Discover Superfoods #3

21 Best Brain-food Berry Recipes

"21 of the best antioxidant-rich berry 'brain-food' recipes on the planet! Help your brain cells ward off dementia and Alzheimer's disease by giving your body the nutritional support it needs to wage a successful battle."

Donna Davidson

Kay Wood

DISCLAIMER

Any references to the health benefits of superfood ingredients in
this recipe book are the opinions of the authors, based on the best data
currently available to them, and are provided for informational
purposes only; they are not intended as medical advice.

If you have an existing medical condition and/or concerns about eating
any of the ingredients mentioned in this book, you should seek the
advice of a qualified medical practitioner before doing so.

* * *

ISBN: 978-0-9941448-1-2

FREE GIFT
FROM DONNA & KAY

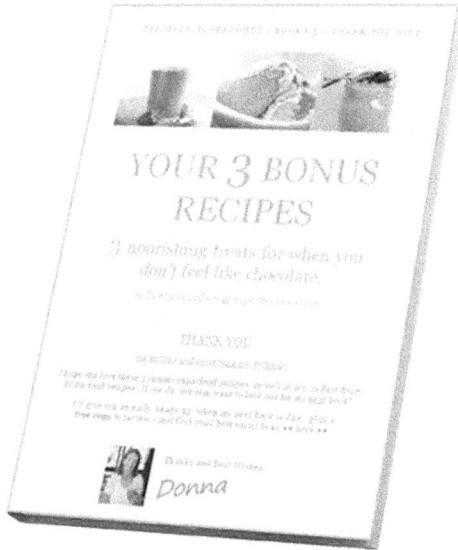

To say thanks for getting our book,
we would like to give you:

3 FREE BONUS RECIPES

'3 Nourishing treats - for when you don't feel like chocolate.'

<< GET YOUR FREE RECIPES HERE >>

Type this into your Internet browser:
superfoodies.co.nz/book3free

* * *

We think you'll <u>like</u> them!

INTRODUCTION:

Here's some
Berry *Good* News

For your brain and general health!

First, the bad news …

- Developing Alzheimer's disease or some other form of dementia is a very real concern for older adults.
- The potential loss of dignity, identity, and independence is a frightening thought for most of us as we advance in age.

Now, the good news …

Berries! Naturally nutritious berries are being shown to hold properties that may provide cellular protection against Alzheimer's disease, age-related memory loss, and other types of cognitive decline.

According to recent research studies conducted at Tufts University in Medford, Massachusetts …

The *flavonoids* found in berries may be able to reverse the cognitive changes and memory problems that usually accompany the aging process. Flavonoids are responsible for many aspects of our brain function. They take part in multiple cellular processes, differing depending on the type of flavonoid involved.

Researcher Fernando Gómez-Pinilla, PhD, studies the effect of nutrition on the brain at UCLA. He explains that flavonoids play important roles in repairing damage in the brain. They do this by influencing how neurons 'talk' to each other and by increasing levels of antioxidants and anti-inflammatory compounds that reduce damage to cells in the brain.

- That's why I created these powerful berry recipes for this, my 3rd book, '21 Best Berry Brain-food Recipes'.
- This book contains 21 of the best superfood berry recipes to help us slow the ageing process and retain mental sharpness, as we get older.

If you enjoyed my first two books on Superfood Cacao (organic chocolate) Recipes (Book #1), and Superfood Smoothie Recipes (Book #2), then you'll definitely enjoy this one too.

Help your brain cells ward off dementia and Alzheimer's disease by giving your body and brain the nutritional support they need to wage a successful battle.

Eating right and boosting your immune system can really make a difference as to:

- How your brain functions
- How you digest and absorb vital nutrients
- How your cells replenish themselves
- Whether you are able to resist debilitating diseases and chronic conditions as you age

Not to mention all the other wonderful general health benefits that berries provide. See Health Benefits of Berries >> pg.48

That's why I created the 21 powerful berry 'brain-food' recipes in this book …

The delicious superfood berry recipes in this book are high in antioxidants and have the proper balance of super nutrition that our ageing bodies need to ward off premature loss of brain function and degeneration of the bodily organ functions that are vital to maintaining our general health and mental acuity.

While nothing can stop you from one day having to bow to the rigours of aging, why not help your body hold on to your mental powers and cognitive abilities, and enjoy robust health for as long as possible?

That's *my* plan any way.

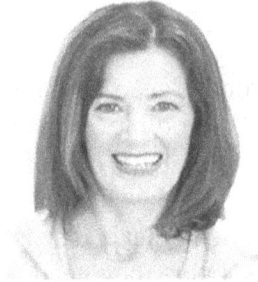

Your Berry Good Health,

Donna

Donna Davidson
January, 2017.

PS. My new philosophy is to 'use food as medicine' – and to use it right NOW. I don't want to be using drugs and / or invasive surgery later in life when I'm suffering from health issues that could have been prevented or delayed by good nutrition and exercise.

Some people complain that healthy foods usually cost more – sometimes a *lot* more. They are right. It is something I really wish I could change, but it isn't within my power to fix at the moment. In the meantime, I suggest that we consider the money we spend on good nutrition *now* to be an investment in maintaining and retaining our good health. I believe the money we spend now is saving us even more money on huge medical bills in the future. Once you lose your health, paying for expensive drugs or surgery becomes a necessity rather than an option.

By thinking of it that way, you can feel better about investing in your future health. Consider that it may be saving you more money down the line; AND you get to enjoy better health in the present so you can live your life to the fullest for as long as possible.

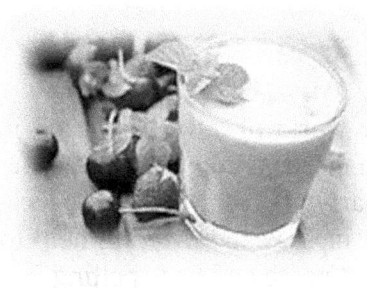

"The flavonoids found in berries may be able reverse the cognitive changes and memory problems that usually accompany the aging process."

–Donna.

Meet the Authors ...

Donna Davidson

Living happily by the Pacific Ocean in beautiful New Zealand, Donna's primary passion has always been in the health, fitness and well-being arena. Several years ago, while working in the superfoods industry, Donna personally experienced the profound benefits of incorporating superfoods into her regular diet and she now credits them with ... Read more on pg.52

Kay Wood

Originally from the world of advertising and marketing, Kay has more recently specialised in copywriting and content creation for the Internet. For nearly 10 years Kay has been 'ghost-writing' info blogs for online businesses and offering help to clients struggling to turn their awkward prose and bad spelling into simple and easily understood ... Read more on pg.57

Meet the Berry Brain-foods ...

Top 10 Health Benefits of Berries

There are loads of berry benefits, but here's our Top 10: Berries carry a high level of antioxidants that are essential to keep our cells healthy and free from life threatening diseases. Our bodies alone cannot produce enough antioxidants to neutralize the harmful free-radicals that invade our healthy cells. Free radicals not only cause disease but ... Read more on pg.48

What are Superfoods?

Superfoods are a special category of foods found in nature. These foods are superior sources of the anti-oxidants and essential nutrients that our bodies need, but cannot make themselves. Superfoods are calorie-sparse and nutrient-dense, so they pack a lot of punch for their weight and deliver ... Read more on pg.60

Superfoods Descriptions + Info

Sacha Inchi Protein Powder: Vegetable protein powder from the South American Sacha Inchi seed. Contains 60% complete protein, all essential amino acids as well as the omega essential fatty acids. Easily digestible and light nutty flavour. Perfect for pre and post workout smoothies, maintaining … Read more on pg.62

Testimonials about Superfoods

Lost over 7kg and feeling so much better: Thank you so much for the healthy delicious treats for Christmas. (See pg.8 of our first book, '21 Best Superfood Cacao Recipes'.) I am still enjoying my new eating regime with super foods. I have lost over 7kg and feeling so much better in myself … Read more on pg.66

Meet the Real Proof …

Will, so-called, 'superfoods' really help me become healthier and feel better? Consider the vital relationship between our modern diet and our health: the steady and observable decline in health and rise of chronic conditions such as allergies, asthma, and skin conditions in western countries over the last 60-100 years is generally agreed, by scientists and … Read more on pg.81

Try the Chocolate Pudding Challenge …

The proof is in the pudding.

In our experience, most people find after adding superfoods to their regular diet (often by simply replacing breakfast with a 'superfood smoothie') that they feel more energetic, start noticing improvements or even the elimination of … Read full 'Chocolate Pudding Challenge' on pg.84

* * *

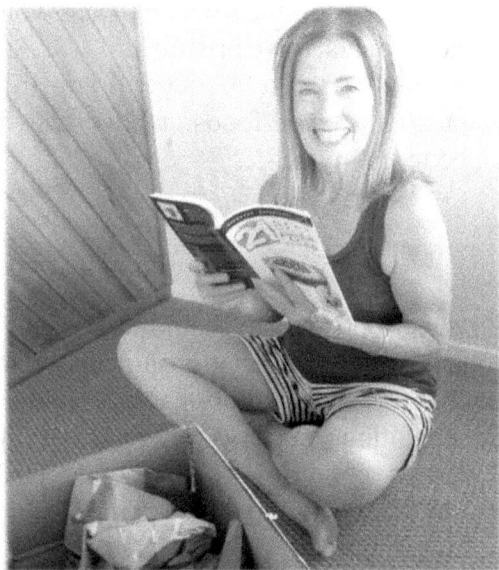

Dreaming of writing your own book?

Many people spend years wanting to write a book but never do … Why?

How did _we_ manage it?

We found a great online writers group, called 'Self-Publishing School'.
They provided coaching, training, support, and a step-by-step plan
to publishing our first book in 90 days, guaranteed.

They also showed us how to format, upload, and successfully market
our book. They involved us in a supportive Facebook community
of fellow writers who gave immediate feedback and positive
advice all along the way. We had a great experience, and
our first two books made it to No.1 on Amazon,
so we happily commend SPS to you.

If you believe you have a book in you, but need
a little help giving birth to it, check out the
Self-Publishing School at the link below:

Self-Publishing School -
http://superfoodies.co.nz/sps

PHOTO Opposite left: The joy of a new author seeing her book in print for the first time!

ACKNOWLEDGMENTS

Special Thanks to ::

The Self-Publishing School gang, especially
Chandler Bolt and Sean Sumner. Without your
amazing coaching and easy step-by-step plan, this book
would probably never exist. We are indebted to you.

We totally recommend Self-Publishing School ::
http://superfoodies.co.nz/sps

Photo Contributors :: Jess Thomson, Donna Davidson
Graphic Design, Layout, Copywriting :: Kay Wood
Recipe Creation + Testing :: Donna Davidson
Mobi/ePub Formatting :: Jay Syder

Published by ::
Super Healthy Kiwi Publishing

Contact the authors by Snail Mail ::
SuperFoodies NZ
267a Harbour Road
Ohope Beach 3121
New Zealand

Email :: info@ superfoodies.co.nz
Website :: http://superfoodies.co.nz
Facebook :: facebook.com/superfoodies.co.nz

Table of Contents

WHERE TO START?

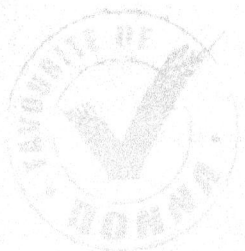

TRY ME!

Not sure which recipe to try <u>first</u>?

They all look good, right?

We have made it easy for you. We'll give you a 'tick start'.
The above tick icon appears next to 3 recipes
personally recommended by Donna.

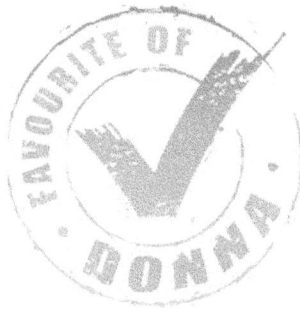

Donna's <u>Top 3</u> 'Tick Start' Recipes:

1. **Strawberry Oats** — TRY ME on pg.14
2. **Berry Buckwheat Porridge** — TRY ME on pg.10
3. **Strawberry Chocolate Mousse** — TRY ME on pg.46

You can't go wrong. It's as easy as 1-2-3!

"So, do yourself a huge favour; grab your ingredients
and easily whip up the healthiest, most delicious
berry brain-food recipes you've ever tasted."

−Donna.

*[If you need to order ingredients it'll take longer, but please don't
let that side-track you from taking this simple first step
on your berry superfood journey to better health.]*

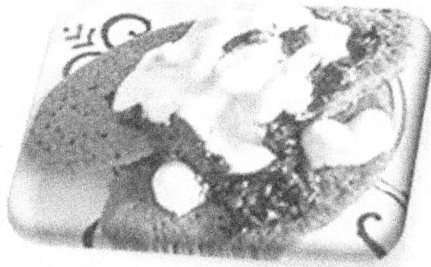

SECTION A

BERRY

BREAKFAST

brain-food

recipes

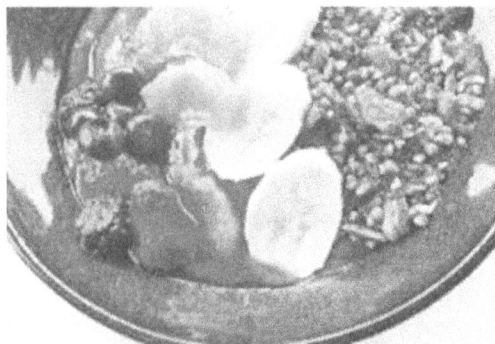

A1. Acai Berry Breakfast Bowl

Serving size: makes 1 bowl
Time to make: 5 minutes

Ingredients

1 tablespoon acai berry powder
1 tablespoon chia seeds
1 teaspoon lucuma powder
1 teaspoon sacha inchi powder
1 cup frozen berries – blueberries / strawberries / or your choice
¾ cup almond milk / or oat milk / milk of choice / or coconut water
1 banana

Method

1. Place all ingredients in blender and blitz until you have a smooth creamy texture like a very thick smoothie you need to eat with a spoon.
2. Place your acai berry breakfast foundation mixture in a bowl.
3. Add granola, nuts and seeds, fresh fruit / or coconut yoghurt.
4. Top with your favourite berries ie. goji berries, strawberries, blueberries.

* Notes:

The taste of Acai is often described as a 'fruity red wine flavour with chocolate overtones'.

Acai has long been revered for its high levels of antioxidants, unique structures of anthocyanins for cellular protection and phytochemicals believed to lower cholesterol. Acai is recognised as one of the world's highest ORAC (Oxygen Radical Absorption Capacity) foods. ORAC measures how well antioxidants neutralise free radicals. It is the free radicals that can harm us, age us and are believed to cause cancer.

Acai has more than twice the antioxidants of blueberries, and nearly ten times those of grapes. The Acai Berry is a low sugar fruit and has one of the lowest glycaemic loads of any fruit. This makes Acai Berry powder ideal for those on a low sugar diet.

If you don't have lucuma powder, you can double up on the sacha inchi / or vice versa.

NEXT Berry Breakfast recipe:
| A2 | Acai Berry Hotcakes | Pg.4

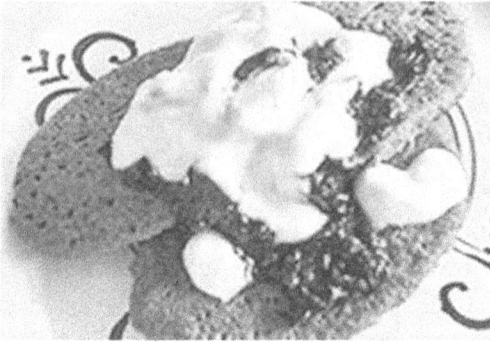

A2. Acai Berry Hotcakes

Serving size: makes 9 hotcakes
Time to make: 30 minutes

Ingredients for hotcakes

2 teaspoons acai berry powder
1 tablespoon lucuma
¼ cup chia seeds
1 cup of whole buckwheat
1-2 teaspoons baking powder
1 pinch of salt
1¾ cups filtered water

Ingredients for berry sauce

1 cup frozen or fresh boysenberries
3 prunes
1-2 teaspoons acai berry powder

Hot cakes Method

1. Place all ingredients except water in blender and start
   processing on low speed.

2. Gradually add water while processing and then blitz to a smooth creamy batter.
3. Heat a non-stick frying pan. Use a little coconut oil to wipe pan if preferred.
4. Ladle batter into frying pan in heaped tablespoon measurements.
5. Cook hotcakes a couple of minutes until small holes appear then turn over in pan to cook other side. These hotcakes are easy to turn over.
6. Put aside and keep warm until ready to eat.

Berry sauce Method

1. Place berries and prunes in saucepan on top of stove.
2. Heat on low heat until prunes are very soft and berries collapsed.
3. Remove from heat and mix until prunes are blended and berries are broken up.
4. Finally mix in acai berry powder and beat to preferred consistency.
5. Serve hotcakes with this antioxidant charged berry sauce and some coconut yoghurt.

* Notes:

Start the berry sauce first so that the berries are slowly condensing while you make the hotcakes. This is a high protein, antioxidant charged breakfast.

NEXT Berry Breakfast recipe:
| A3 | Antioxidant Granola | Pg.6

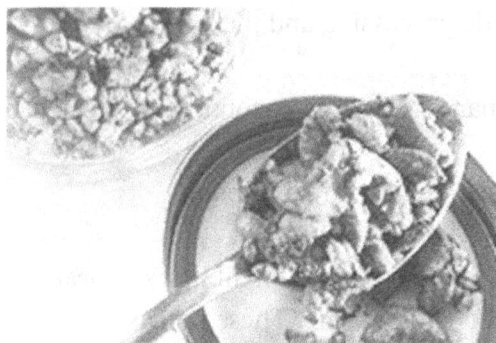

A3. Antioxidant Granola

Makes: one large jar full / or about 10 servings
Time to make: 10 minutes + 30 minutes cook time

Ingredients

2 cups buckwheat groats - hulled buckwheat / or use rolled oats
½ cup cashew pieces / or almonds
½ cup walnuts
½ cup pumpkin seeds
½ cup sunflower seeds
1 teaspoon cinnamon
1 teaspoon vanilla extract / or vanilla paste
1 grated orange rind (grated skin from one orange)
3 tablespoons maple syrup / or honey
¼ cup cranberries
¼ cup goji berries
2 teaspoons each of acai berry powder / or maqui berry powder /
or camu camu powder

Method

1. Heat the oven to 100 degrees.

2. Place the first six ingredients in a bowl, buckwheat, cashews, walnuts, pumpkin and sunflower seeds, cinnamon.
3. Add the orange rind and stir to mix through.
4. Warm the maple syrup so it is easy to pour, add the vanilla and pour over the dry ingredients.
5. Cover two oven trays with baking paper, halve the mixture and spread evenly over the two trays.
6. Place in oven and bake for approximately 15 minutes. Remove from oven and stir the granola before returning to the oven. After another 10 minutes check the granola it may be almost done. It can be over-done very quickly.
7. Remove from oven and allow to cool on the trays.
8. When cold, mix in the cranberries and goji berries, as well as the acai berry powder, maqui berry and camu camu powders.
9. Store granola in a large air-tight jar or container.

* Notes:

The granola goes a very dark colour because of the maple syrup, but be careful not to overcook it. This granola is exceptionally delicious, I found myself picking while I was photographing it.

The combination of the berry powders and goji berries makes it a very potent antioxidant brew. It is such a delicious gluten free granola to impress your guests with. Serve with fresh berries and coconut yoghurt.

NEXT Berry Breakfast recipe:
| A4 | Banana Berry Pancakes | Pg.8

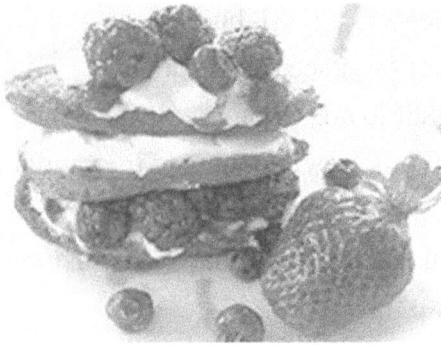

A4. Banana Berry Pancakes and Berry Oats

Serving size: makes 6-8 pancakes
Time to make: 20 minutes

Ingredients

2 teaspoons maqui berry powder
1 tablespoon lucuma powder
1 tablespoon chia seeds
1 cup almond meal (ground almonds)
1 teaspoon gluten-free baking powder
1 teaspoon cinnamon
2 eggs
½ cup almond milk
2 ripe bananas mashed to smooth pulp
Berries, coconut yoghurt, and maple syrup to serve

Method

1. Mix the mashed bananas and eggs together. This can be done by hand or in a blender or food processor.
2. Add all remaining ingredients: maqui berry powder, chia seeds, lucuma, almond meal (ground almonds), baking powder, cinnamon and almond milk.

3. Blend together well by hand or blitz in the blender.
4. Add more almond milk if required so that mixture is not too thick.
5. Allow mixture to rest for a couple of minutes.
6. Heat a pan over low heat and add a little coconut oil.
7. Spoon pancake mixture into rounds onto the pan and shape as desired.
8. Cook on low heat for about 5 minutes then flip over and cook on the other side. Don't be tempted to turn up the heat.
9. Serve pancakes with berries, coconut yoghurt and maple syrup according to taste.

* Notes:

These pancakes are much lighter in texture than my buckwheat hotcakes. It is so easy and quick to whip up for a treat with friends. Another delicious way to appreciate the health benefits of berries.

NEXT Berry Breakfast recipe:
| A5 | Berry Buckwheat Porridge | Pg.10

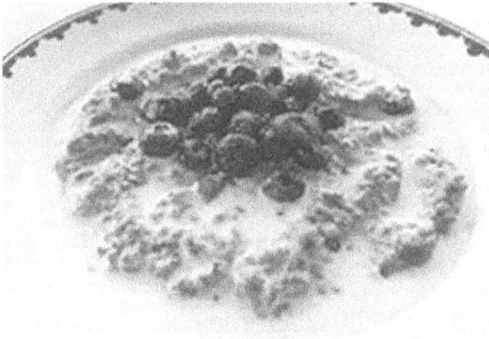

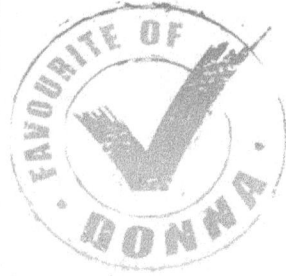

A5. Berry Buckwheat Porridge

Makes: 2 servings
Time to make: 10 minutes + overnight soaking

Ingredients

1 tablespoon maqui berry powder / or acai berry
2 tablespoons chia seeds
½ cup toasted hulled buckwheat (groats)
1 teaspoon vanilla paste
½ teaspoon cinnamon powder
2 cups almond milk / or milk of your choice
1 handful of chopped dates / or dried fruit of your choice
1 cup frozen blueberries
Coconut milk to serve

Method

1. Start preparation the night before.
2. Toast the buckwheat groats in a dry pan in a single layer on a med to high heat. Swirl the pan at regular intervals to toast groats evenly, takes about 5 mins.
3. In a bowl place the toasted buckwheat, chia seeds, vanilla, cinnamon, dates and milk. Stir well, rest a couple of minutes then stir again.

4. Cover bowl and place in refrigerator overnight for the buckwheat to soften.
5. Also the night before place frozen blueberries in a bowl, sprinkle with maqui berry powder and allow berries to defrost on the bench overnight.
6. In the morning place the buckwheat porridge in a saucepan and cook over low heat for 5 mins, stirring frequently.
7. Stir the defrosted berries so the maqui berry is infused. Pour half the berries into the cooked porridge and stir.
8. Pour the porridge into a breakfast bowl and top with the remaining berries and coconut milk.

* Notes:

This porridge sounds like a lot of fuss but it is really quick and easy. Toasting the buckwheat is essential, because it creates the delicious unique flavour - and I find toasting the groats before going to bed is very relaxing.

Buckwheat is gluten-free; it is a seed, not a wheat. With a low glycaemic rating and good quality protein it will sustain your energy for longer; not to forget all the vital minerals it contains. The combination with the berries is truly delicious and another way to maximise your antioxidant uptake. The maqui berry powder enhances the flavour of the blueberries.

I find this porridge doesn't stick to the bottom of the saucepan, so it saves on washing up time too. Very important!

NEXT Berry Breakfast recipe:
| A6 | Four Seed Berry Breakfast | Pg.12

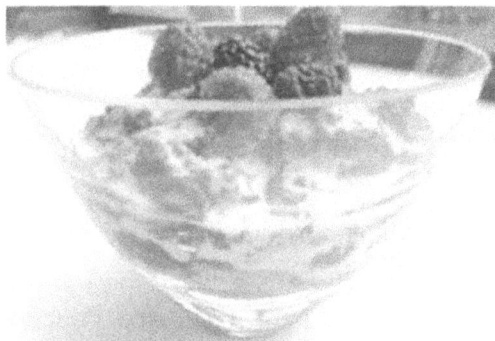

A6. Four Seed Berry Breakfast

Serving size: makes 2 servings
Time to make: 5 minutes + soaking time overnight

Ingredients

2 teaspoons maqui berry powder
1 tablespoon chia seeds
1 tablespoon linseeds
1 tablespoon sunflower seeds
1 tablespoon pumpkin seeds
1 tablespoon desiccated coconut
1 teaspoon vanilla extract
½ cup filtered water / or milk of your choice
1 tablespoon maple syrup
1 cup coconut cream / or yoghurt
2 helpings of mixed berries and fruit of your choice

Method

1. Place the first eight ingredients in a bowl and mix thoroughly with a spoon.
2. Cover and place in refrigerator overnight, alternatively stand for at least 1 hour.

3. In the morning take the seed mixture out of the fridge and mix with a spoon.
4. Take 2 clean bowls and layer, beginning with the seed mix on the bottom.
5. Cover bottom layer with berries then cover again with the seed mix.
6. In between layers swirl some maple syrup and coconut cream / or yoghurt.
7. Finish by topping with a layer of berries.

* Notes:

This is so quick and easy because the ingredients only need to be measured out and soaked overnight. All ingredients are usually easily found in a health conscious pantry, so they are easy to put your hands on!

NEXT Berry Breakfast recipe:
| A7 | Strawberry Oats | Pg.14

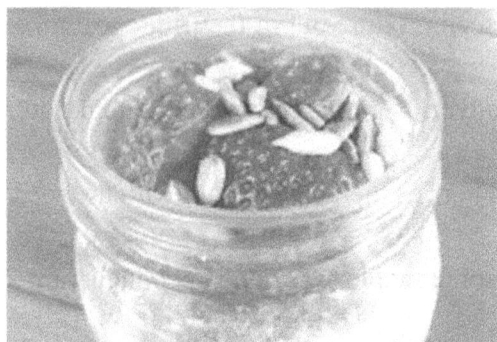

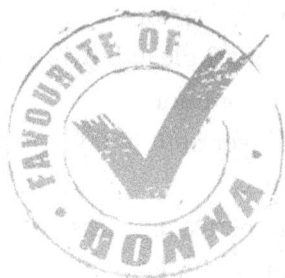

A7. Strawberry Oats

Serving size: makes 2 servings
Time to make: 5 minutes + overnight soak time

Base Ingredients

2 tablespoons chia seeds
1 cup of rolled oats
2 tablespoons desiccated coconut
1 teaspoon vanilla extract
1 teaspoon cinnamon powder
2 cups milk (almond milk with coconut milk is a good combination)

Strawberry Topping Ingredients

2 teaspoons maqui berry powder / or acai berry powder
1 punnet of strawberries
1 tablespoon honey, maple syrup / or date paste
Toasted sunflower seeds to garnish

Base Method

1. Take 2 jars with screw tops.
2. Halve the base ingredients and place in the 2 separate jars.

3. Screw the tops on the jars and shake well to mix.
4. Leave for 15 minutes then give jars another good shake so the chia seeds don't clump together.
5. Place in refrigerator overnight.
6. In the morning remove from refrigerator and combine with strawberry topping.

Strawberry Topping Method

1. Take 4 strawberries and cut into quarters.
2. Place remaining strawberries and honey in blender and blitz until a pureed consistency.
3. To assemble, place 1 teaspoon of maqui berry powder in each jar on top of the base.
4. Pour half the strawberry puree on top and with a long spoon stir to mix through.
5. Then add the remaining half of strawberry puree and the strawberry quarters on top and decorate with toasted sunflower seeds.

* Notes:

This is a very easy and quick berry breakfast that tastes and looks decadently good. It doesn't have to be made in jars, but I find it a convenient way to take breakfast with me if I have an early start somewhere. You can 'up' the antioxidants with more berry powders if you want.

NEXT: Section B | Berry Smoothie recipes | Pg.17

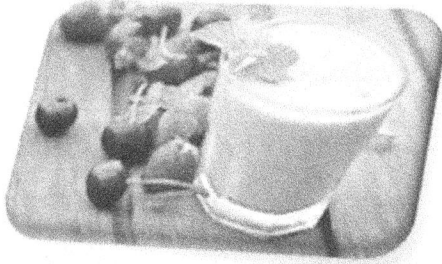

<u>SECTION B</u>

BERRY

SMOOTHIE

brain-food

recipes

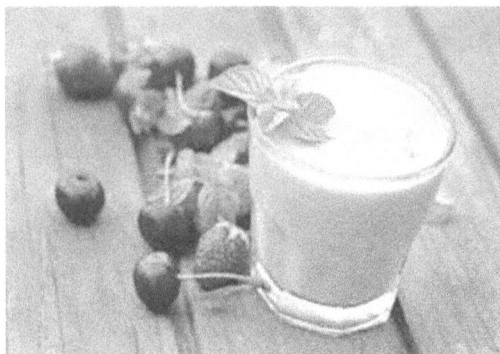

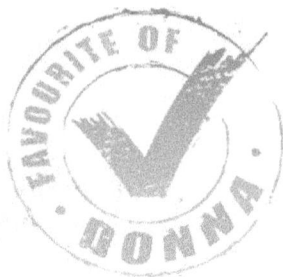

B1. Berry Cocktail Smoothie

Serving size: makes 2 smoothies
Time to make: 10 minutes

Ingredients

1-2 cups fresh mixed berries / or frozen berries

2 frozen chopped bananas - skin removed

1 handful of fresh mint leaves

2 limes - juice and flesh - peeled

2 cups of filtered water / or coconut water

2 teaspoons maqui berry powde r / or acai berry powder

1 tablespoon sacha inchi protein powder

1 tablespoon lucuma powder / or yacon powder

Method

1. Place banana, mint leaves, lime juice and flesh, in the blender
    with some of the water - and blitz until well processed.

2. Add the berries, maqui berry powder, sacha inchi and lucuma,
    along with the remaining water.

3. Blitz to a smooth texture.

4. Pour into glasses and enjoy.

* Notes:

The limes and mint add a very fresh twist to this delicious berry smoothie. I know you will enjoy this one.

NEXT Berry Smoothie recipe:

| B2 | Berry Goji Smoothie | Pg.20

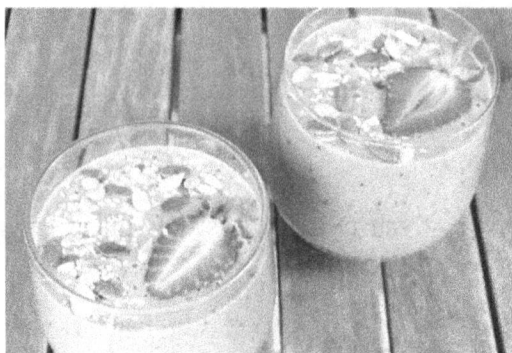

B2. Berry Goji Smoothie

Serving size: makes 2 smoothies
Time to make: 10 minutes

Ingredients

2 cups fresh / or frozen mixed berries
2 large oranges
2 tablespoons goji berries
2 cups of filtered water / or coconut water
2 teaspoons maqui berry powder / or acai berry powder
1 tablespoon sacha inchi protein powder
1 tablespoon lucuma powder
1 tablespoon chia seeds
½ teaspoon of vanilla paste / or vanilla extract

Method

1. Peel and chop oranges leaving some white pith on.
2. Place all ingredients into a blender.
3. Blitz until all the fresh fruit is processed to a smooth texture.
4. Pour into glasses and enjoy.

* Notes:

Goji berries have all the essential amino acids and have a deserved reputation as an anti-aging food. I love the taste of them, especially together with orange.

Allow a few minutes for the dried berries to rehydrate - the flavour is more intense that way.

NEXT Berry Smoothie recipe:
| B3 | Blueberry Smoothie | Pg.22

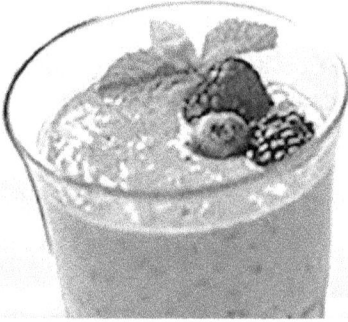

B3. Blueberry Smoothie

Serving size: makes 2 smoothies
Time to make: 10 minutes

Ingredients

1-2 cups fresh / or frozen blueberries
2 frozen chopped bananas - skin removed
2 cups almond milk / or milk of your choice / or coconut water
2 teaspoons maqui berry powder / or acai berry powder
1 tablespoon sacha inchi protein powder
1 tablespoon lucuma powder
1 tablespoon chia seeds

Method

1. Place all ingredients into a blender.
2. Blitz until all the fresh fruit is processed to a smooth texture.
3. Pour into glasses and enjoy.

* Notes:

According to Dr Oz (from the 'Dr Oz Show' on TV), lucuma is an 'energy stabilizer'. Since lucuma has a very low glycaemic index, this is a logical conclusion. Blueberries naturally are higher in fruit sugars than other berries so lucuma is a great companion to the other ingredients in this smoothie.

NEXT Berry Smoothie recipe:
| B4 | High Antioxidant Berry Smoothie | Pg.24

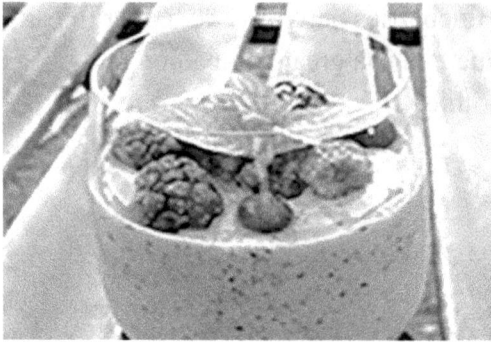

B4. High Antioxidant Berry Smoothie

Serving size: makes 2 smoothies
Time to make: 10 minutes

Ingredients

1 cup mixed fresh / or frozen berries (blueberry, blackberry, raspberry or your own combination)
1 frozen banana chopped - skin removed
½ cup fresh pineapple
2 cups almond milk / milk of your choice / coconut water
2 teaspoons maqui berry powder / or acai berry powder
2 tablespoons sacha inchi protein powder
1 tablespoon chia seeds

Method

1. Place all ingredients into a blender.
2. Blitz until all fresh fruit is processed to a smooth texture.
3. Pour into glasses and enjoy.

* Notes:

If you don't happen to have fresh berries available, you can double the maqui berry or acai berry powders. It makes this Berry Smoothie very convenient to prepare when travelling.

You can also add 2 teaspoons of our fermented greens powder to aid digestion and boost the nutrient uptake.

NEXT Berry Smoothie recipe:
| B5 | Pomegranate Berry Delight Smoothie | Pg.26

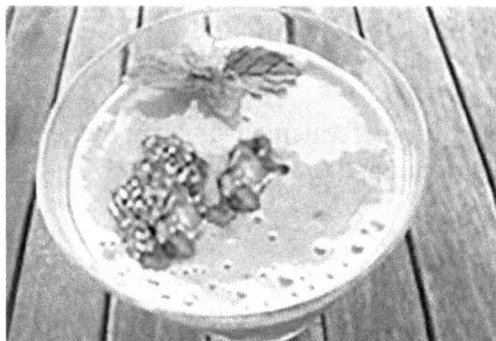

B5. Pomegranate Berry Delight Smoothie

Serving size: makes 2 smoothies
Time to make: 10 minutes

Ingredients

1 cup fresh / or frozen raspberries
1 cup fresh / or frozen blueberries
1 cup pomegranate seeds
1 frozen banana – skin removed
6 medjool dates / or 8 dried chopped dates
2 cups filtered water / or coconut water
1 tablespoon sacha inchi protein powder
1 tablespoon maca powder
2 teaspoons acai berry powder

Method

1. If using dried dates, let them soak a few minutes in some of the water.
2. Place dates, frozen banana and water into a blender.
3. Blitz until well processed.
4. Add raspberries, blueberries, pomegranate seeds, sacha inchi,

maca and acai berry powder to blender; then blitz until well processed and smooth.

5. Pour into glasses and enjoy.

* Notes:

Pomegranates are new for me but I am totally fascinated with them, now that I've learned how to easily remove the seeds. (I treat it like a lemon, cut in half and squeeze or use a lemon squeezer.)

There is not a lot of reliable nutritional information on pomegranates, but their colour alone tells us it is high in antioxidants. This means they are good for heart health and cellular protection.

Protein powder is an important element in smoothies: it helps carry the sugars to even out the glycaemic load. Protein supports our immune system, our metabolism, and helps our bodies to sustain lean muscle.

NEXT Berry Smoothie recipe:
| B6 | Strawberry Date Surprise Smoothie | Pg.28

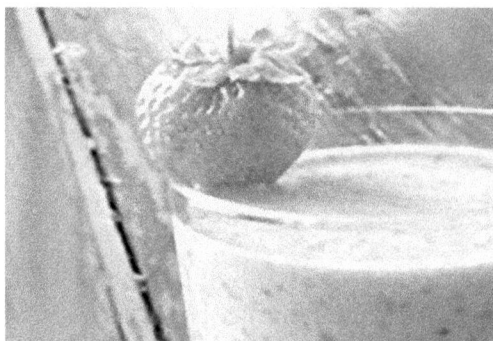

B6. Strawberry Date Surprise Smoothie

Serving size: makes 2 smoothies
Time to make: 10 minutes

Ingredients

2 cups fresh / or frozen strawberries

2 cups spinach washed and stalks removed

6 medjool dates / or 8 dried chopped dates

2 cups filtered water / or coconut water

1 tablespoon sacha inchi protein powder

2 tablespoons lucuma powder

1 teaspoon camu camu powder

Method

1. If using dried dates, let them soak a few minutes in some of the water.
2. Place spinach, dates and water into a blender.
3. Blitz until well processed.
4. Add strawberries, sacha inchi, lucuma and camu camu then blitz until well processed and smooth.
5. Pour into glasses and enjoy.

* Notes:

This is a vitamin C charged smoothie with no citrus fruit needed. Strawberries are high in vitamin C and camu camu is an extremely potent vitamin C berry.

Lucuma contains beta-carotene to support the immune system making this smoothie a good marriage for fighting the flu.

Protein powder is an important element in smoothies - it helps carry the sugars to even out the glycaemic load. Protein supports our immune system, our metabolism and helps our bodies to sustain lean muscle.

NEXT Berry Smoothie recipe:
| B7 | Strawberry Fields Smoothie | Pg.30

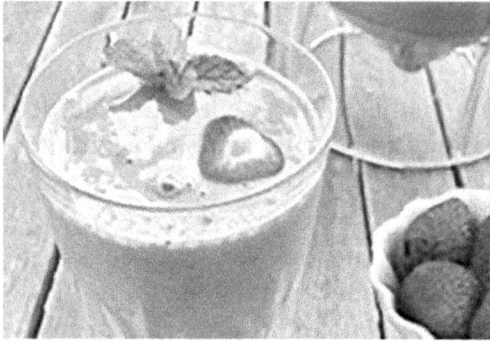

B7. Strawberry Fields Smoothie

Serving size: makes 2 smoothies
Time to make: 10 minutes

Ingredients

2 cups fresh / or frozen strawberries
2 frozen bananas chopped - skin removed
2 large cups almond milk / or milk of your choice / or coconut water
2 teaspoons maqui berry powder / or acai berry powder
1 tablespoon maca powder
2 tablespoons lucuma powder

Method

1. Place all ingredients into a blender.
2. Blitz until all the fresh fruit is processed to a smooth texture.
3. Pour into glasses and enjoy.

* Notes:

Strawberries are a low calorie food high in vitamin C and manganese. They are a good detoxifier.

I love maca powder because it's not only delicious, but it also supports the thyroid gland.

However, maca powder is a product that a few people may initially have a small physical reaction to it. This reaction usually presents as minor stomach cramps. Most people have no problems at all, but I want you to be fully aware just in case you are the exception.

If you are not used to maca powder, try using only a teaspoon at first, then increase it gradually if you have no reaction to that quantity.

NEXT: Section C | Berry Treats recipes | Pg.33

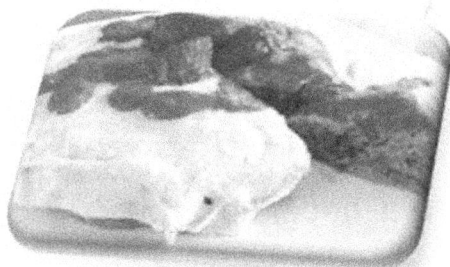

SECTION C

BERRY

TREATS

brain-food

recipes

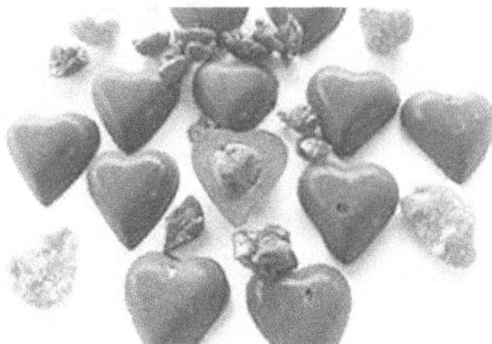

C1. Acai Berry Chocolates

Makes: 36 chocolates
Time to make: 15 minutes

Ingredients

30g cacao butter
$\frac{1}{3}$ cup cacao powder
2 teaspoons acai berry powder
3 tablespoons virgin coconut oil
½ teaspoon vanilla extract
1 tablespoon brown rice syrup / or maple syrup
Dried fruit for chocolate centres

Method

1. Place cacao butter and coconut oil in a heatproof glass jug.
2. Place jug in a bowl of boiling water so the butter and oil melt to liquid.
3. Take jug out of boiling water and add the remaining ingredients, cacao powder, acai powder, brown rice syrup and vanilla. Beat with a whisk.
4. When well blended take a tray of chocolate moulds and place a piece of dried fruit in the centre of each chocolate mould.

5. Pour the chocolate over the fruit and fill the moulds.
6. Place the tray in refrigerator or freezer for chocolates to set.
7. Chocolates should set in the freezer in approximately 30 minutes.
8. Remove tray from freezer and pop the chocolates out onto a serving plate.

* Notes:

These chocolates melt easily so keep them in the refrigerator whenever possible.

There is no limit to the flavours you can create. I used dried strawberries and cranberries for the centres and sometimes threw in some goji berries.

The combination of the acai berry powder and cacao powder gives these chocolates a very high antioxidant status.

NEXT Berry Treats recipe:
| C2 | Acai Berry Parfait | Pg.36

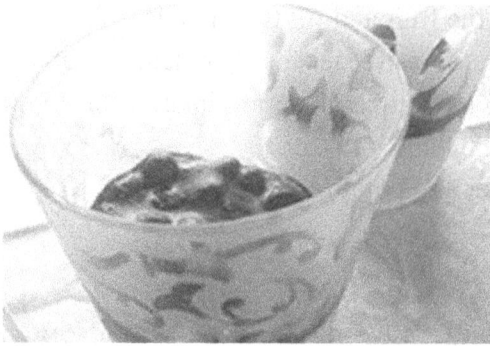

C2. Acai Berry Parfait

Serving size: makes 2 servings
Time to make: 20 minutes

Base Ingredients

1 cup cashew nut pieces
1 cup filtered water
1 tablespoon honey
2 teaspoons agar powder (vegetable gelatin)

Acai Berry Topping Ingredients

½ cup frozen / or fresh blueberries
2 teaspoons acai berry powder
1 tablespoon honey
2 teaspoons arrowroot / or tapioca flour
½ cup filtered water

Base Method

1. Blitz cashew nuts in blender till fine powder.
2. Add remaining base ingredients to blender and blitz altogether until very smooth.

3. Pour mixture into small saucepan and heat until thickened, stirring regularly.
4. Pour into 2 serving glasses and leave to cool in refrigerator.

Acai Berry Topping Method

1. Heat blueberries in a pot until defrosted or heated through.
2. Mix the arrowroot, water and honey in a cup and pour over the berries.
3. Keep stirring until you have a nice thick texture.
4. Stir in Acai berry powder and pour over the base ingredients.
5. Place in refrigerator to cool for at least 30 minutes.

* Notes:

Look after your guests with this healthy delicious dessert. Very quick and easy to prepare and loaded with goodness.

You could use any berries for the topping but don't forget to add a quality acai berry or maqui berry powder for an extra boost of antioxidants for cellular protection.

NEXT Berry Treats recipe:
C3 Boysenberry Muffins | Pg.38

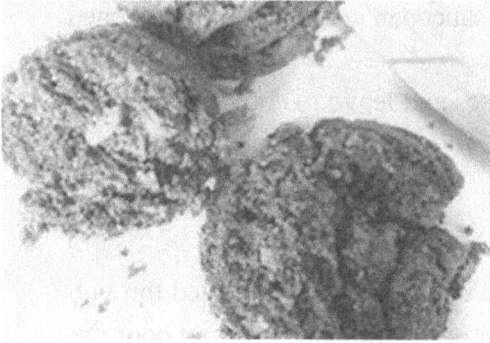

C3. Boysenberry Muffins

Serving size: makes 6 large muffins
Time to make: 10 minutes + 35 minutes cook time

Ingredients

1 cup boysenberries
½ raw apple - finely chopped into little pieces.
1 tablespoon lucuma powder
2 teaspoons maqui berry powder / or acai berry powder
1 teaspoon cinnamon
1 teaspoon lecithin (optional)
1-2 teaspoons baking powder
1½ cups almond meal (ground almonds)
1 pinch of salt
2 eggs
30ml melted coconut oil
1 tablespoon honey / or maple syrup

Method

1. Heat oven to 170C / 340F.
2. Place all dry ingredients in a large mixing bowl.
3. Add coconut oil, honey and eggs.

4. Mix to a smooth batter.
5. Fold in berries and apple.
6. Spoon into 6 paper cups / or patty tins.
7. Bake in oven for 35-40 minutes.

* Notes:

These muffins are light and moist to eat, high in protein and antioxidant rich. They are also delicious; that's my opinion as 'not usually a muffin person'.

NEXT Berry Treats recipe:
| C4 | Maqui Berry White Chocolate | Pg.40

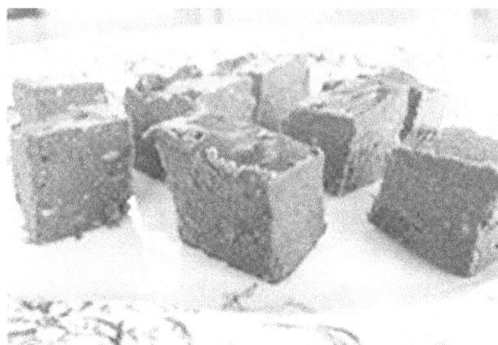

C4. Maqui Berry White Chocolate*

Makes: 60 pieces
Time to make: 30 minutes

Ingredients

2 heaped tablespoons maqui berry powder
1 tablespoon lucuma powder
200g cacao butter
½ cup coconut butter
½ cup coconut cream
½ cup maple syrup
2 teaspoons vanilla essence
1 teaspoon lemon juice
¼ teaspoon fine Himalayan salt
1½ cups cashew nut pieces

Method

1. Blitz cashew nuts in blender or food processor till fine powder.
2. Melt cacao butter in glass jug resting in a bath of boiling water.
3. Soften coconut butter.
4. Add all ingredients to a food processor and blitz until the mixture is well blended and very smooth.

5. Pour into 26 x 19 cm cake tin lined with baking paper.
6. Place in refrigerator or freezer to set. After about 15 minutes, test firmness and cut into pieces before it sets too hard.
7. Return to refrigerator to set completely.

* Notes:

The coconut butter can be replaced with a good coconut oil. I often make my own coconut butter by blitzing 2 cups of desiccated coconut in the food processor for about 10 minutes.

It is quite an arduous process scraping the coconut down the sides of the food processor as you go along, but it is a very economical way to make coconut butter.

* Yes, it _is_ white chocolate! The darker colour in the picture is because it has taken on the purple hue of the the maqui berry powder. So don't be surprised when your 'white' chocolate turns out to be purple! You haven't got the wrong recipe.

NEXT Berry Treats recipe:
C5 | Raspberry Cake | Pg.42

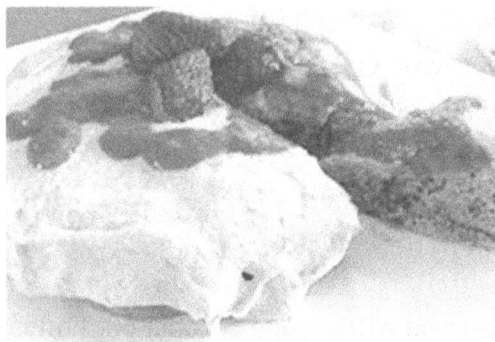

C5. Raspberry Cake

Serving size: makes 8-12 servings
Time to make: 15 minutes + cook time 45 minutes
+ 10 minutes for the cashew cream

Cake Ingredients

1 tablespoon lucuma powder
1 cup frozen / or fresh raspberries
½ cup coconut flour
2 teaspoons gluten-free baking powder
⅓ cup liquid coconut oil
2 tablespoons maple syrup / or honey
1 teaspoon of vanilla bean paste
6 eggs

Cashew Cream Topping Ingredients

1 cup cashew nut pieces
½ cup filtered water
½ teaspoon vanilla bean paste
1 teaspoon camu camu / or maqui berry powder - to sprinkle on top
1 handful of berries to garnish

Cake Method

1. Preheat oven to 160 C / 320 F.
2. Whip the eggs, maple syrup and vanilla with a beater until light and creamy.
3. Pour in the coconut oil while still whipping and mix well.
4. Add the coconut flour, lucuma and baking powder, mix until well combined.
5. Fold in the defrosted raspberries.
6. Pour mixture into an 18cm round cake tin. Best to first line the tin with baking paper.
7. Bake for 45 minutes / or until cake is cooked through.
8. Cool for 30 minutes before removing cake from tin to cool completely.
9. When completely cool garnish with cashew cream and berries.

Cashew Cream Topping Method

1. Place cashew nut pieces in blender and blitz until fine powder.
2. While blender is going pour in the water and vanilla, then blitz very well until delicious creamy texture forms. Continue to blitz some more to make sure it is smooth.
3. Let stand in the refrigerator to set a little.
4. When manageably firm spread over the cake.
5. Decorate with fresh berries and sprinkle camu camu powder / or maqui berry powder on top.

* Notes:

Use defrosted frozen berries / or fresh berries for the top. The sprinkle of camu camu or maqui berry powder enhances colour whilst boosting your antioxidant intake.

NEXT Berry Treats recipe:
| C6 | Raspberry Popsicles | Pg.44

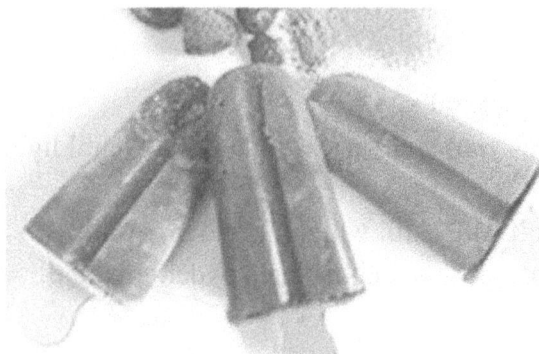

C6. Raspberry Popsicles

Serving size: makes 8 popsicles
Time to make: 5 minutes + 2 hours freezing time

Ingredients

1 cup raspberries - fresh / or frozen
1 banana - skin removed
2 teaspoons maqui berry powder / or acai berry powder
1 tablespoon lucuma powder
1 tablespoon sacha inchi protein powder
1 tablespoon date paste / or a few dates soaked for 15 minutes in some water
2 cups almond milk / or water

Method

1. Place all ingredients into a blender.
2. Blitz until a smooth texture appears.
3. Pour into ice block moulds with sticks and freeze until set hard.

* Notes:

This recipe is so quick and easy. Perfect for children, as well as adults. I had originally intended to add some maple syrup but when I tasted it I found there was no need. It has a big berry flavour and ample natural sweetness.

Nutritionally packed with protein and antioxidants; these popsicles are such a pleasurable, but highly nourishing, snack.

NEXT Berry Treats recipe:
C7 | Strawberry Chocolate Mousse | Pg.46

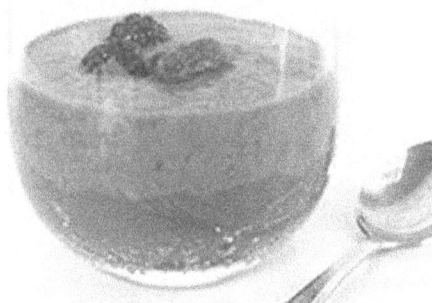

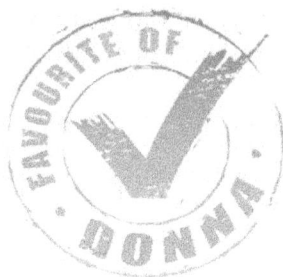

C7. Strawberry Chocolate Mousse

Serving size: makes 2 servings
Time to make: 20 minutes

Base Ingredients

3 tablespoons cacao powder
2 teaspoon lucuma / or yacon powder
½ cup raw cashew nut pieces
1 tablespoon date paste
1 pinch of salt
¼ cup filtered water
1 chopped banana fresh / or frozen – skin removed

Strawberry Topping Ingredients

1 cup fresh / or frozen strawberries
1 tablespoon date paste
1 teaspoon yacon powder
1 teaspoon freeze dried camu camu powder

Base Method

1. Place cashew nuts in blender and blitz until a fine powder.

2. Add remaining dry ingredients with some of the water to blender, also add the banana and the date paste, then blitz until smooth and creamy.
3. Adjust the consistency with the water remaining.
4. When well processed spoon chocolate mousse into base of mousse glasses.
5. Refrigerate while you make the strawberry topping.

Strawberry Topping Method

1. Place strawberries in blender. If using frozen berries, allow to thaw slightly.
2. Add date paste, yacon and camu camu powders.
3. Blitz until smooth, be careful not to over process.
4. Remove glasses from refrigerator and top with the strawberry topping.
5. Garnish as you desire.

* Notes:

To make a date paste I finely chop dried dates and cover with hot water to soak and soften. Leave overnight / or for just one hour / then blitz to a paste in food processor. The paste can be stored in the refrigerator for a few days.

This Strawberry chocolate mousse is easy and quick to make. It is light and full of flavour while being extremely antioxidant rich.

NEXT: Health Benefits of Luscious Berries | Pg.48

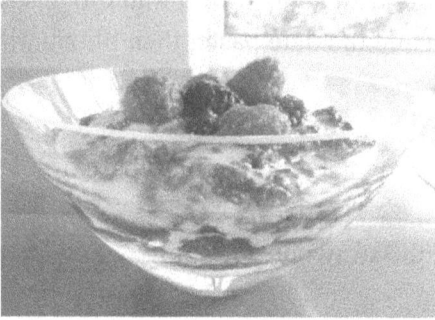

Top 10 Health Benefits - of luscious Berries

There are so many benefits to berries, but here's *our* Top 10:

1. Berries carry a high level of antioxidants that are essential to keep our cells healthy and free from life threatening diseases.

2. Our bodies alone cannot produce enough antioxidants to neutralize the harmful free-radicals that invade our healthy cells. Free radicals not only cause disease but also premature aging. Berries keep our antioxidant levels topped up.

3. Berries are rich in vitamin C which helps to keep the skin firm by aiding collagen production. Collagen strengthens skin and supports elasticity and firmness. For me there is no argument, a healthy vibrant glowing skin is the best apparel to be seen in.

4. Anthocyanins, found in berries are also good for preventing the oxidation of cholesterol. Whether you have high or low levels of cholesterol, the oxidation of circulating cholesterol makes it easier to stick to the walls of your arteries causing narrowing. This build-up of plaque can eventually lead to high blood pressure.

5. It is the flavonoids found in berries that may be the key to reversing the cognitive changes and memory problems that

usually accompany the aging process. Flavonoids take part in multiple cellular processes, depending on the type of flavonoid. They are responsible for many aspects of our brain function.

6. Flavonoids play an important role in repairing damage in the brain. They do this by influencing how neurons "talk" to each other and by increasing levels of antioxidants and anti-inflammatory compounds that reduce damage to cells in the brain. Berries are rich in flavonoids.

7. Not all berries are equal. Acai berries are a low sugar fruit and have one of the lowest glycaemic loads of any fruit. This makes Acai Berry powder ideal for those on a low sugar diet without any compromise on the antioxidant levels.

8. Berries are rich in Vitamin C as well as Vitamins A, B1, B2, B3 and E and also calcium, magnesium, zinc and copper. With this amazing nutritional profile, it's easy to see that berries can benefit your health, and may help slow the ageing process itself.

9. Berries are relatively low in calories.

10. Lastly, when we eat berries from South America - such as the antioxidant-rich Acai and Maqui berries - we are supporting the regeneration of the Amazon rain forest.

Trees are now being protected in the Amazon basin, rather than being destroyed, because farming the berries is providing alternative incomes for local families.

So, eating these berries, or superfood products made from them is not just good for you, you're helping to save the whole planet too!

* * *

Will these superfood Berry Recipes work for _you_?

Superfoods sceptics will say that there is no 'absolute proof' (yet) that putting all these good things into your body will lead to better health in the long-run. How do I answer that challenge? I say ...

There's one way to know for _sure_ ...

Try superfoods ... then monitor the results for yourself! Superfoods obtained from a reputable source will be natural, nutrient-rich, and uncontaminated by chemicals and preservatives; unlike most of the foodstuffs you consume every day from your local supermarket. Trying them for a reasonable period of 2-3 months should reveal whether they will deliver the benefits that I and others claim to receive. This would be similar to your doctor trying a medication for a period to see if it works for you. However, if you have any concerns about taking superfoods you should get your doctor's 'go ahead' to try them, first.

Mainstream ...

Mainstream medical professionals (apart from surgeons, physical therapists, and psychological counsellors) mainly seem to focus on drug-based _solutions_ to health problems; and they usually come with a long list of potential 'side-effects' and legal disclaimers.

The bottom line of the small print boils down to the fact that 'you are choosing to take this drug at your own risk' and, having been warned, don't think you can sue the drug company if it all goes horribly wrong.

My Experience ...

My experience (along with a wealth of anecdotal evidence) of superfoods is that I _feel_ better, my brain seems to work better, and medical conditions, that I couldn't find an answer for using traditional medicine (drugs), went away.

Balance ...

Of course, you need to approach superfoods (like anything else) in a balanced and sensible way. So, if one superfood smoothie makes you feel better, don't drink ten of them! It won't be 10 times better for you. In fact, it would be bad for you. Just like abusing caffeine or alcohol. Or anything.

Common sense ...

Your body has natural tolerances and can only absorb certain amounts of anything each day. That's why many of the vitamins included in supplement capsules are often wasted, passing through your body without being absorbed. It's worth consulting your doctor and getting a blood test to see if you are actually deficient in anything. Together you can make an informed decision about if supplements will help, or if any deficiencies cab be better supplied by improving your daily diet. I prefer the dietary solution because it's not only safer but could save you flushing money, literally, down the toilet. A few simple changes to your eating habits may be an easier fix and be much better for you in the long run.

Drugs v. Natural ...

As I get older, having experienced both sides of the equation in trying to keep my brain and body healthy, I prefer the natural approach in my daily life. It is working for me.

I believe, adding a daily dose of nutrient-rich superfoods to your diet will work for you too.

It might even change your life.

Donna Davidson

- January, 2017.

* * *

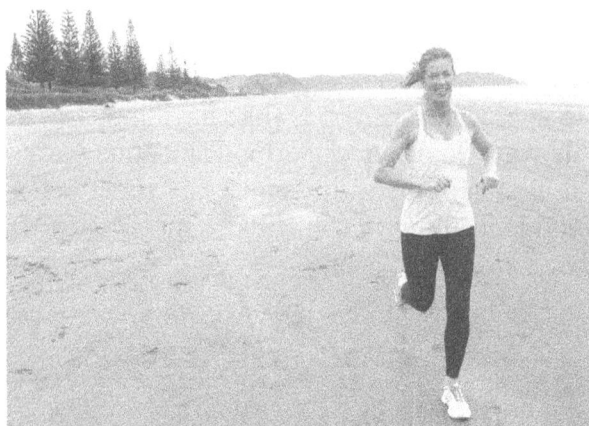

Donna Davidson Biography

- Author, business woman, recipe creator, 'superfoodie'.

Living happily by the Pacific Ocean, in New Zealand's beautiful North Island, Donna's primary passion has always been health, fitness and well-being.

Donna began her fitness career as an aerobics instructor; after receiving her diploma from Lords Gym in Perth, Australia, she trained at Jane Fonda's Workout Studio in Beverly Hills, California.

After establishing her own fitness studio back in Auckland, New Zealand, Donna was chosen to teach aerobics to New Zealand's Americas Cup yacht squad, as part of a new fitness and motivational program preparing them, for their first Americas Cup challenge.

Later, while working in the superfoods industry, Donna experienced the profound benefits of adding superfoods to her regular diet. She now credits superfoods with helping her conquer 2 major health challenges in her life; dangerously high blood pressure and 'cyclic vomiting' syndrome.

Donna also realized that she had much more energy, and increased mental acuity.

Wanting to *share* her discoveries with like-minded people, she decided to found her own superfoods company and online store; with the 'modest' aim of teaching as many people as possible about the benefits of superfoods, and making it easy for them to obtain them online.

The result was superfoodies.co.nz, which she created with the help of her friend, Kay Wood. Her goal was simple: to source the highest-quality superfood products and teach simple, sensible, delicious ways for ordinary folks to enjoy their health benefits - without any hype or exaggeration.

Donna's first superfoods recipe book, '21 Best Cacao (Natural Chocolate) Recipes' was launched in November, 2015 and quickly became an Amazon best seller – reaching the #1 spot several times!

The second book in Donna's 'Discover Superfoods' series, '21 Best Superfood Smoothies', contains 21 delicious ways to drink yourself to better health through nutrition. It is already getting rave 5 Star (the highest) reviews.

Now, you are reading Donna's third book, '21 Best Brain-food Berry Recipes' delivers 21 of the best antioxidant-rich berry 'brain-food' recipes on the planet!

These superfood berry recipes are especially designed by Donna to help your brain cells ward off dementia and Alzheimer's disease by giving your body and brain the nutritional support they need to wage a successful battle.

Eating right and boosting your immune system can really make a difference as to how your brain functions, how you digest and absorb vital nutrients, how your cells replenish themselves, and whether you are able to resist debilitating diseases and chronic conditions as you age.

You've made a great choice to invest in your health and well-being by obtaining this book. Please let us know your results and experiences. Be sure to reach out to Donna and her *Superfoodies* team, if you need any help or advice.

* * *

EMAIL Superfoodies :: info@superfoodies.co.nz
FOLLOW on Facebook :: Facebook.com/SuperFoodies

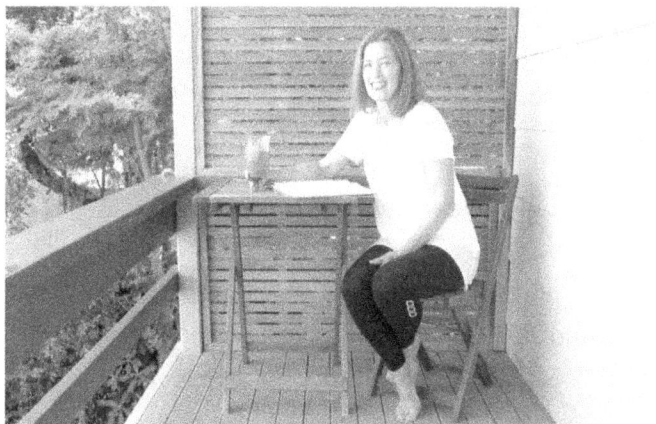

Donna's High Cholesterol story in her own words ...

"Despite a strong sporting background and regular fitness regime, I still battled debilitating health issues earlier in my life, for which I couldn't seem to find an answer.

Quite by accident, the answer came when I landed a job in the superfoods industry; I experienced increasingly positive changes by adding specific superfoods to my daily diet.

Prior to that, I had been diagnosed with 'cyclic vomiting' syndrome. This meant that, approximately once a month, I would throw up continuously over 24 hours - which just wiped me out physically. Shortly after I started having a green superfood smoothie every morning this vomiting cycle completely disappeared.

I realized that my daily green smoothie was alkalising my digestive system and setting me up for the day. A second (unexpected) consequence was the rapid reduction of my bad cholesterol.

I have always been very fit and slim, so I'd been totally shocked to find my cholesterol was at a dangerous level. Although my mother had suffered from angina, and died with dangerously high cholesterol, aged 64, I had always considered myself 'fit and healthy' (despite my vomiting problem) and it had never occurred to me that I could be susceptible too.

After 3 months of drinking my green smoothie, my cholesterol went from 7.3 to 4.8. The result not only wowed *me*... but they *stunned* the nurse reading them out to me over the phone! I kept my printed test result sheets to prove to myself that I hadn't dreamt it, because even *I* couldn't believe it for ages. It took time to really sink in. I think, because it was literally life-changing for me.

To write the books in my 'Discover Superfoods' series I've had to draw deeply from all the knowledge I gained over 7 years of working in the superfoods industry; in order to create some of the best, easy-to-make, health-giving, superfood recipes available.

These recipes will help you add loads of wonderful superfoods to your normal diet - in a variety of ways - that are not just super-nutritious and delicious, but often down-right decadent.

Please share your experiences with me, or ask me any questions you may have. I'd love to hear from you."

Donna Davidson
- Revised, January, 2017.

* * *

FOLLOW Donna on Facebook :: Facebook.com/SuperFoodies
EMAIL Donna :: info@superfoodies.co.nz

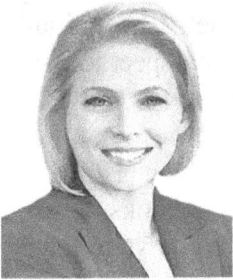

Kay Wood Biography

- Author, blogger, copywriter, web marketer, 'superfoodie'.

Originally from the world of advertising and marketing, Kay has more recently specialised in copywriting and content creation for the Internet. She also adores anything Tolkien, especially Hobbits.

For nearly 10 years Kay has been 'ghost-writing' info blogs for online businesses and offering her help to clients struggling to turn their awkward prose and bad spelling into simple and easily understood information about their products and services.

Kay and Donna became friends while working together to create Donna's superfoodies.co.nz website, in late 2013. Kay also worked closely with Donna to help her realise her ideas for the 'look and feel' of her superfood product packaging and the 'Superfoodies' logo design.

Kay and Donna found themselves 'clicking' as a team during that creative process. They both shared a common desire to present in an honest and balanced way the genuine health benefits to be gained by incorporating superfoods into one's diet - while at the same time dialling back some of the hype surrounding superfoods.

Kay's story in her own words ...

"When I suggested to Donna that putting together some of her favourite and most delicious superfood recipes into a cookbook 'might be a good idea', to help show people how many ways superfoods can be incorporated into their diet, she initially hesitated because it sounded like such a daunting prospect to cover all, or even most, of the major superfoods in one book.

I later modified the original idea, suggesting to Donna that she should create a series of short, practical recipe books sharply focused on only one superfood in each book, pared down to the 21 absolute best recipes that Donna could come up with.

We both agreed that cacao would be the perfect superfood for book #1 - because everyone loves chocolate right? And healthy, or certainly healthier, ways to enjoy chocolate have got to be a great addition to any chocolate lover's recipe book collection.

So, with me cracking the whip and Donna creating, making, baking, eating and perfecting the recipes, our first book, '21 Best Superfood Cacao Recipes', was born.

Then came book two: '21 Best Superfood Smoothie Recipes'. Everyone loves a delicious smoothie, right? Even the kids! (Pssst! Parents, don't tell them they're healthy!) And these smoothies are packed with all the wonderful nutrients often lacking in today's over-processed supermarket offerings or nullified by chemicals and preservatives. See Donna's own story and read some of our testimonials to see what a powerful difference one morning superfood smoothie can make to your life!

And now our third baby (kind of), '21 Best Berry Brain-food Recipes'! These recipes are powerful weapons to help your brain cells ward off dementia and Alzheimer's disease by giving your body and brain the nutritional support they need to wage a successful battle.

Finally, a huge thanks for buying our book!

Please use it and really benefit from it. I mean that sincerely. Good intentions (without action) just pave the pathway to health hell.

You won't regret the time and trouble you invest in making these recipes when you discover the benefits for yourself and how amazingly delicious they are! I think they are Donna's best yet!

Kay Wood

Living in Aotearoa / New Zealand / Middle Earth / with the Hobbits.

- Revised, January, 2017.

PS. If you love these recipes and /or start to notice real health improvements, please don't forget to give us an honest review on Amazon. That really helps us spread the word to all those who still don't know there are natural superfood alternatives to junk food. Thank you.

* * *

What are Superfoods?

Superfoods are a special category of foods found in nature: these foods are superior sources of the essential nutrients and antioxidants that our bodies need, but cannot make themselves.

Superfoods are calorie-sparse and nutrient-dense, so they pack a lot of punch for their weight and deliver more of what our bodies need in one go. Foods that have been elevated to superfood status in recent years include those rich in antioxidants, vitamins, minerals, essential fatty acids, including omega-3 fatty acids.

Contrary to what some people wrongly believe, Superfoods are NOT nutrition created through advancements in food sciences. They are actually looking back to nature for what it does best: providing us with amazing and complex combinations of nutrients, beautifully balanced to supply us with what our bodies require to flourish.

This is simply going back to the wild and harnessing foods in their natural forms, with all their benefits intact. It is celebrating nature's wealth of nutrients in all its varieties. We have within our reach a true powerhouse of natural ingredients to provide us with the nutrition we need for healthy living.

Many superfoods are unique to their own geographical position in the world and this is usually because their local environment was perfect for producing them. Fortunately, in our modern world of advanced communication, travel and cultural appreciation, we are currently discovering an abundance of nutrient-rich superfoods we have previously never heard of. e.g. superfoods from South America, like the sacha inchi seeds, maqui berries, maca root, lucuma, and camu camu.

See Superfood Descriptions on pg.62 of this book, for more info.

There is no official definition of a superfood, and the EU has banned the use of the word on packaging, but that hasn't stopped many food brands from funding academics to research the health benefits of their products. Nor does it deter the health conscious from seeking and following eating regimes abundant with good nutrient-dense foods that they enjoy and feel the benefits of.

Superfoods can be processed under 40 degrees Celsius without damaging their nutritional profile and being classed as 'raw foods'. This makes storage and availability more convenient and versatile. e.g. superfood powders for smoothies and snacks are generally dried below 40 degrees Celsius.

An awareness of the kinds of foods that we're now calling 'superfoods', has been increasing rapidly over the last few years. Along with a better appreciation for how the foods we consume affect our bodies, as well as our long-term health.

We're also finding ourselves being 're-introduced' to many of the foods that were well-known to past generations, yet have been neglected for decades. We have lost touch with the knowledge of plants and natural compounds that our supposedly more primitive ancestors used to survive and heal themselves, before drugs were invented.

This is a knowledge that we all need to re-discover – if only to balance out the modern reliance on artificial drug based treatments. We're not saying that all drugs are bad, but returning to a lot of the effective yet natural ways of maintaining and restoring our health can't be a bad thing, either.

That way we can save drugs for serious health problems that require sudden, dramatic intervention. Thus, we may actually increase their efficacy and, by reducing their usage, also reduce the risk of creating drug resistant bacteria and the instances of harmful side-effects. Our immune systems will also thank us. Drugs often weaken our immune systems by killing the pro-biotic bacteria in our gut, interfering with the body's ability to digest food properly.

* * *

Superfoods Descriptions + Info

These are the dried superfoods Donna uses in her recipes:

Sacha Inchi protein powder: Vegetable protein powder from the South American Sacha Inchi seed. Contains 60% complete protein, all essential amino acids, as well as the omega essential fatty acids. Easily digestible and light nutty flavour. Perfect for pre/post workout smoothies, to maintain and build muscle.

More about Sacha Inchi powder + where to buy it :
Type into your web browser: www.superfoodies.co.nz/des-a

Maqui Berry powder: Reported to have the highest antioxidant/anthocyanin content than any other fruit or berry. Grows wild in the patagonian rain forests of Chile and Argentina. Contributes to cardiovascular health, cellular protection against oxidative stress, immune support and detoxification. Maqui berry powder is deep purple in colour and has a delicious rich berry flavour.

More about Maqui Berry powder + where to buy it :
Type into your web browser: www.superfoodies.co.nz/des-b

Acai Berry powder: Like maqui berry powder, acai has a very high antioxidant content with unique structures of anthocyanins for cellular protection and phytochemicals believed to lower cholesterol levels. Contains high levels of vitamin E and essential fatty acids to support clear smooth skin. Acai is low in sugar, deep purple in colour and perfect for smoothies and breakfast recipes.

More about Acai Berry powder + where to buy it :
Type into your web browser: www.superfoodies.co.nz/des-c

Lucuma powder: Comes from a fruit native to the Peruvian Andean region. It provides beta-carotene known for immune support as well as calcium phosphorous and iron for energy. It has a low glycaemic score of around 25 while it imparts a natural sweet, creamy, citrusy, maple flavour.

More about Lucuma powder + where to buy it :
Type into your web browser: www.superfoodies.co.nz/des-d

Maca powder: Contains unique alkaloids known to stimulate the hypothalamus and pituitary glands which in turn improve the overall functioning of the endocrine system responsible for balancing hormones. Grown in Bolivia and Peru it has a vanilla/nutty taste which is very appealing in smoothies. Although one of the most popular and consumed superfoods it is a food that can make some people feel queasy or have stomach cramps, but this is not common. I recommend small doses to start with e.g. 1 teaspoon in a smoothie, working up to 1 tablespoon per day.

More about Maca powder + where to buy it :
Type into your web browser: www.superfoodies.co.nz/des-e

Yacon powder: A natural sweetener containing high levels of inulin a fructooligosaccharide that provides sweetness in a form that is indigestible by humans so they do not affect blood sugar levels and simply pass through the digestive tract to be eliminated. Since these sugars are not digested and also low in calories they are suitable for use in diet and low calorie foods.

More about Yacon powder + where to buy it :
Type into your web browser: www.superfoodies.co.nz/des-f

Yacon syrup: The same as yacon powder, it's GI is only ONE. I find this syrup delicious in recipes, cacao drinks and smoothies. It is the perfect substitute for maple syrup if you are watching your sugar intake, often not easy to find and unfortunately a little more expensive.

More about Yacon syrup + where to buy it :
Type into your web browser: www.superfoodies.co.nz/des-g

Camu Camu berry powder: The camu camu berry from the Amazon region is presenting higher levels of vitamin C than any other fruit tested to date. Latest results are showing 56 times more vitamin C than Lemons. It is a potent addition for any smoothie.

More about Camu Camu berry powder + where to buy it :
Type into your web browser: www.superfoodies.co.nz/des-h

Blueberry powder: Well known for its antioxidants and anthocyanins. It also contains resveratrol also found in grapes which has been linked to heart health. A convenient powder to add flavour to smoothies.

More about Blueberry powder + where to buy it :
Type into your web browser: www.superfoodies.co.nz/des-i

Chia seeds: A must have ingredient for a superfood pantry. When added to smoothies they make you feel full and satisfied for longer periods.Chia seeds contain more omega 3 fatty acids than salmon. They are low glycaemic and are another source of protein.

More about Chia seeds + where to buy it :
Type into your web browser: www.superfoodies.co.nz/des-j

Fermented greens powder: A powerful formula which acts as a natural probiotic because of the good bacteria produced from the fermentation process. This natural probiotic aids digestion, assists absorption and has many healing functions. It is my personal MUST HAVE in a morning smoothie to set me up for the day.

More about Fermented greens powder + where to buy it :
Type into your web browser: www.superfoodies.co.nz/des-k

Cacao powder: Cacao powder has an extremely high antioxidant score on the ORAC scale. By eating high antioxidant foods in our diet it is believed we are helping to guard against cellular and tissue damage which often lead to serious illness.

Magnesium is abundant in Cacao Powder and it is magnesium that is known to be the most important mineral for a healthy heart. Cacao is a mood elevator due to the presence of serotonin.

More about Cacao powder + where to buy it :
Type into your web browser: www.superfoodies.co.nz/des-l

Cacao butter: Is the ingredient that sets chocolate and other chocolate treats. It contains oleic acid which is the same healthy fat found in olive oil. It also is a good source of vitamin E. It does not need to be stored in the refrigerator. It melts to liquid at 35 degrees Celsius.

More about Cacao butter + where to buy it :
Type into your web browser: www.superfoodies.co.nz/des-m

Cacao nibs: Has a similar nutritional profile to cacao powder. Nibs are the shavings and fragments from the cacao bean. They add crunch and texture to chocolate treats and smoothies.

More about Cacao nibs + where to buy it :
Type into your web browser: www.superfoodies.co.nz/des-n

* * *

Superfoods Testimonials

These are a few typical examples of unsolicited testimonials and comments about superfood products from happy customers who purchased from Donna's own website: superfoodies.co.nz

Lost over 7kg and feeling so much better ...

"Thank you so much for the healthy delicious treats for Christmas. I am still enjoying my new eating regime with super foods. I have lost over 7kg and feeling so much better in myself. Everyone comments on how well I look and that my skin is glowing. Coming along to your sugar free cooking class was the best thing I have done in a long time." – **Kate.**

* * *

My husband is really noticing the benefits ...

"Nick, my husband has been using the green smoothie powder and really noticing the benefits – he is a landscaper so needs the energy - plus he has sinus problems and this has really helped with that as well. Brilliant." – **Annemarie.**

* * *

Helping me cope with the stresses of my current life ...

"Still going strong with the smoothies and have one most days. Really like them and I think they are helping me cope with the stresses of my current life – very sick husband, work, coping with ten staff, visitors and the rest of the daily grind. They fill me up now that I add soy or almond milk until the next meal and I have found that my sweet tooth has dissipated to a large degree – not wanting something sweet every day, which is a real bonus. So all good, and all thanks to you!" – **Sigrid.**

* * *

I'm 'regular as clock-work' – without medication … wahoo!

"I'm pleased to tell you that I am having a smoothie every morning and my Green Smoothie Shot and the great thing is, I have been able to stop taking the Laxsol tablets that I have had to take for years. I decided to stop taking them straight away because they aren't life threatening (just uncomfortable if it didn't work) to see if the Chia seeds and Green Smoothie Shot made any difference immediately and I'm pleased to say it has, and I've never been able to go off these tablets before, so now I'm 'regular as clock-work' and without medication … wahoo!

Now for the extra good news, **I have lost 2kgs in just under 2 weeks** of using the Chia Seeds, Cacao Powder and Green Smoothie Shot - so the products are obviously cleansing my body well. I'm using all natural 100% pure coconut water in my smoothies and a frozen banana which is awesome." – **Michele.**

* * *

Immediately noticed an increase in my energy and general wellbeing …

"At last I can get a fermented probiotic greens powder (Donna's Green Smoothie Shot) in New Zealand! I have been searching high and low for a fermented greens powder in New Zealand since I moved here some years ago. When living in Sydney I was introduced to this product and I immediately noticed an increase in energy and general wellbeing – I was overworked and I truly think that this is what helped keep me going. When I left Australia I took as much with me as I could carry in my case, but that is long gone and I have been missing it ever since.

So thank you 'SuperFoodies.co.nz' for bringing this wonderful product to New Zealanders – it is every bit as good as I remember!" – **Xenia.**

* * *

I have already made <u>double-lot</u> of Choc Fudge protein bars …

"Thank you very much for yesterday, I so enjoyed it. Have already made 'double-lot' of Choc Fudge protein bars and my children like them!" – **Hiria Wallace.**

* * *

Enhanced well-being and energy (and we didn't get sick) …

"My husband and I have just returned from a month's trip around Morocco and every morning we took "Green Smoothie Shot" without fail. We were pleasantly surprised we did not experience any sickness and felt this product enhanced our well-being and energy to make the most of our holiday." – **Yvonne Porter.**

* * *

I learnt so much and changed my eating already …

"I learnt so much and have changed a few things with my eating already. Would love to carry on learning more." – **Jodeen Mitchell.**

* * *

You are so passionate about healthy food …

"Thanks ladies! You're both awesome. Very inspiring, as you are both so passionate about healthy food. Will try recipes out on my family." – **Jeanette Pleijte.**

* * *

Read more Testimonials
superfoodies.co.nz/category/testimonials/

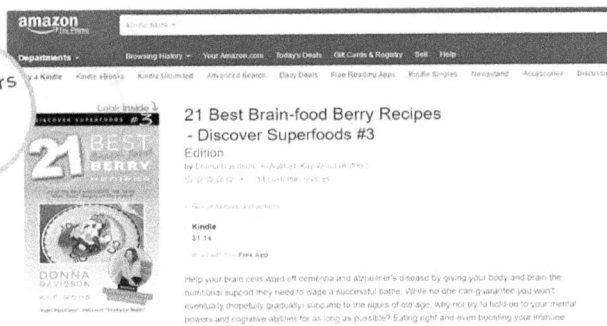

What our readers think of this book!

21 Best Brain-food Berry Recipes - Discover Superfoods #3 Edition

★★★★★ 5 Star Amazon Book Reviews:

- "An everyday go-to cookbook for those serious about eating for maximum health."

- "My favourite is the Raspberry Popsicles ... I could have them every day."

- "The way to good health can be fun, invigorating, nutritious and very easy!"

- "As a Health and Fitness Coach, I thought I had tried it all ... not even close! These recipes opened up my mind to so much I'd been missing out on."

- "Thank you Donna for writing this book. I work with women who have breast cancer and I can finally refer them to a cook-book that is in alignment with everything I have been teaching about healthy eating. Thank you!"

- "I love berries! My kids do too! I am constantly looking for unique and out of the box ways to prepare healthy meals for my family. I am so happy I found this gem!"

- "The recipes in this book all look delicious, and I'm looking forward to trying them. First up will be 'Strawberry Oats'."

See more reviews here   www.amazon.com/dp/B01LWJLKOD

WHERE TO START?

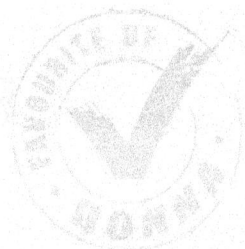

TRY ME!

Isn't 'fresh' always best?

And other Frequently Asked Questions, like:

1. What are all these superfood powders and dried processed products?
2. Isn't fresh always best?
3. What makes them 'super' foods - as opposed to ordinary foods?
4. How do these dried processed superfoods compare with fresh foods that are also called superfoods?
5. Are all these powders and dried stuff really superfoods?
6. Where can I get all these fancy dried superfood products?
7. Do they sell them in my local supermarket or do I have to go to a Health Food Shop?

* * *

If *you've* asked any of these questions … here are the answers, according to Donna and Kay:

QUESTION: "So, why are you using 'dried' superfood powders and products in these recipes?"

KAY'S ANSWER: This is something that often seems weird to people unfamiliar with using the dried forms of superfood products that are now available on the market.

In an ideal world, we would all have acai berries, maqui berries, blueberries, bananas, and cacao growing fresh in our backyards and we would pick them at the height of their potency and use them fresh every day.

Sadly, no matter where you live, this would be practically impossible. Either for climatic reasons, soil suitability, time poverty, lack of backyard garden space, lack of knowledge about how to actually grow and maintain these kinds of plants, and a zillion more reasons.

Even the supposedly 'fresh' fruits and vegetables we have available locally vary in nutritional value and taste, because of rising population numbers, they have to be grown quickly, picked, preserved, transported, displayed, and sometimes artificially enhanced to look appealing to consumers. The average 'fresh' tomato that most modern city dwellers eat is vastly different to the 'fresh' tomato that our grandparents or great-grandparents would have eaten. I remember my father growing tomatoes and strawberries in our small town New Zealand backyard and how 'gobsmack-ingly' delicious they were compared with the bland equivalents I purchase from the supermarkets these days.

When the population of the planet was relatively small, a mere 200 years ago, it was possible (at least theoretically) to grow enough food for the whole population of the world on the fertile farmland available, while also allowing enough time for excess land to lay 'fallow' for several years in order for the soil to recover the nutrients sucked out of it by the plants as they grew. That goodness, of course, was transferred to us when we ate those plants. Now, however, with farmland diminishing worldwide and poor farm and land management practices being common in many parts of the world, we already have less farmland available than is required to feed us all. This means that the land is being over utilised, the nutrients being stripped and never replaced, leading to less and less nutrients in the actual fruit and vegetables being grown on that land.

And then there's contamination from chemicals, such as fertilisers and pesticides, pollution, climate change, contamination from poor storage, unhealthy additives, and bad practices engaged in by unethical companies quite happy to put profit before their customers' health.

In an ideal world, 'fresh' would reign supreme. But in the real world, often the best we can do is combine 'fresh' (hopefully from the least contaminated sources) with high-quality dried nutrient sources - like the superfoods we recommend - in order to give our bodies and immune systems access to nutrients that aren't guaranteed to be in our food anymore.

If you live in a city, and especially if you have a busy, pressurised lifestyle, you probably don't have a garden, or the time to maintain one. My dad knew what nutrients his tomatoes needed and what kind of things were bad for them. Even though I ate his produce with glee, I never acquired his knowledge or skills and have never had much of a garden, sadly. Now, I wish I'd taken more notice and been more willing to learn from him.

I am sure the same is true for many people, especially those younger than me; the whole idea of growing things yourself is a foreign concept. For some people even the idea of eating green things is foreign, and they think all food comes in packages that you heat up in a microwave. For those people, on a practical level it would be much easier to throw some dried superfood ingredients into a blender; chop up a few available fruits or vegetables from the supermarket, and blend them all into a delicious smoothie in a couple of minutes, than to contemplate actually growing anything. Never-mind having the land, plants or seeds, tools, fertilisers, knowledge, and the time to actually do it. Not to mention trying to control all the pests without risk to you or the soil. Whoops, I mentioned it!

Is a tropical rainforest growing outside your window?

Many of the wonderful dried superfoods we use are only found in South America - probably because of the peculiarities of that climate and the evolution that occurred there in the isolation of the fertile tropical jungles. We think that buying superfoods from ethically responsible companies - who pick them 'fresh' at exactly the right moment, dry process them within an hour or two of being picked to lock in their nutrient content at its most potent - is a great way to access the tremendous nutrient value they contain.

Some still say, "You can get *everything* you need by eating fresh fruit and vegetables from the supermarket". If you read everything I wrote prior to this, and still believe that's a true statement, then you are entitled to your opinion. Donna and I would respectfully disagree with you. We have seen many people restore their health and well-being, as well as supporting their immune systems to fight and often eliminate stubborn health conditions. This is anecdotal evidence for sure, but, often, anecdotal evidence is only evidence waiting for science to catch up.

We can't guarantee that everybody who tries superfoods will experience the same results, but the same would be true if you visited the doctor and he recommended a course of treatment or certain medications. A doctor will never guarantee you anything. Also, try contacting the drug companies and see if they'll guarantee you that their products will work. Even the ones that have been supposedly approved and double-blind tested.

At the end of the day, as Donna and I often say, the 'proof is in the pudding' and you need to try something for a reasonable period of time and see if it works for you. Of course, you should do your 'due diligence'. Do as much research as you can, reference as much expert opinion as you can, try and find as much testimonial from those who have similar conditions to yourself and see what results they obtained, and then ... you still end up with having to decide whether you will try them to see if they'll work for you.

This would be true of *anything*.

When Donna first tried green smoothies to see if they would help lower her high-cholesterol levels, a few years ago, she never expected them to eliminate her chronic 'cyclic vomiting' problem as well. That was a total surprise. Her life changed completely just because she added a green superfood smoothie every morning! There was no medical solution available at the time. The best she could do was to 'manage' the problem with injections of drugs.

My own experience is less dramatic: I was experiencing stomach pains and just feeling generally fatigued and unwell. When Donna sent me some 'green smoothie shot powder' which I added to a morning smoothie I came right within a week and have felt more balanced and that my stomach and digestion was working as it should. I don't feel queasy and nervous about my gut the way I previously did when it felt unstable and uncomfortable on a regular basis, despite the fact that my diet was comparatively healthy.

I hope my thoughts on the 'why' part of the "*why* do you use these kind of dried products?' question, has helped.

I'll let Donna explain her ideas of the pros and cons between 'fresh versus dried' superfoods, since she has much more expertise, not to mention experience, than me.

Kay Wood
Revised January, 2017.

* * *

'Fresh' vs. 'Dried' Superfoods ...

QUESTION: "How do these dried, processed superfoods compare with fresh foods that are also called 'superfoods'?"

DONNA'S ANSWER: I personally believe in and work with both.

When I'm time poor, I'm grateful to have my stash of dried superfoods in my pantry, so that I can whisk up a delicious and satisfying smoothie and be on my way to take on the day. When I have time to spare and have been fresh produce shopping I enjoy experimenting with produce in season mixed with my superfoods.

I know I can 'bank' on the variety of tastes and nutrition in dried superfoods, and they are as easy as having the stock in my pantry.

Fresh produce is not always at your fingertips, unless you have a prolific garden ... lucky you. So I say, you can 'have it all' by combining the use of dried and fresh (whatever is seasonally available).

* * *

Here are some 'Pros and Cons' - for fresh versus dried:

Fresh is Best - when:

1. You know you are buying or gardening organically.
2. Your produce is harvested at its peak nutritional stage.
3. Your produce is stored in a cool place or refrigerator.

Downside of 'Fresh':

1. Using fresh produce requires lots of your 'TIME' for organisation, storage, planning, and preparation.
2. Seasonal unavailability of your favourites.

Dried is Best - when:

1. They are harvested at their nutritional peak and immediately processed to lock in their nutritional profile.
2. You can safely buy organic and see where the product is from on the label.
3. Storage is more convenient and takes up less space.
4. No produce preparation in the form of cutting, washing etc.
5. Less shopping.
6. Less planning ahead.
7. If you buy from a reputable company, quality and purity is more certain.

Downside of 'Dried':

1. 'Taste' is the only real downside to using dried superfoods.

The huge advantage of dried superfoods is that they are preserved at the highest level of nutrient potency and they degrade very slowly when well stored. But they can't beat the wonderful fresh 'taste' of local seasonal produce.

'Fresh' is delicious and nutritious; offering a wide variety of taste and flavour combinations, depending on the season. Whenever I make a smoothie or design a recipe I never rely solely on the dried superfood products because, although they may be delivering the desired nutritional punch that our bodies and immune systems need so desperately, our taste buds also need to enjoy themselves!

That's why my recipes are full of 'real foods' and 'superfoods', in the forms of fresh fruits, nuts, seeds, and vegetables, as well as dried superfoods. I want the recipes to be a balance between taste and health, so they deliver on both fronts. In previous generations we often believed that if it was good for you it had to 'taste bad' - but these days we expect healthy food to be delicious and delightful to our taste buds, as well.

That's my goal when I sit down to design any new recipe. If I'm modifying an existing recipe, it will be because I can improve either the nutritional content, or the taste factor, or both. That was pretty easy for this book because it's all about smoothie recipes so they weren't too hard to make delicious, or healthy either - as long as you only use quality ingredients.

Please make sure you stick closely to my recipes and resist temptation to add any 'nasties', like extra sugar - or you'll undermine all my good work!

Sometimes, when you're beginning to add superfoods to your diet, your taste buds will need a little time to adjust to the lack of excess sugar and salt and other nasties that your system has been used to.

Don't worry, after a very short time you will begin to enjoy the wonderful variety of natural flavours that were masked by these unhealthy additives in the past. *Then* your taste buds will begin to take you on a voyage of (re)discovery of flavours and taste sensations that you've been missing out on, or not enjoying to their fullest intensity.

Donna

Revised January, 2017.

* * *

Where can I buy these dried superfoods?

If you haven't heard of some of the superfoods (fresh or dried) – like lucuma powder or acai berries, for example - that Donna uses in her recipes, you may be wondering, 'Where may I obtain these weird and wonderful new superfood ingredients?'

1. Health Food and Organic Stores
2. Pharmacies / Drug Stores
3. Specialty Food Shops
4. Some Supermarkets – ask at your local supermarket
5. Websites – order from local businesses online
6. Amazon.com – or your country's Amazon website
7. Google – search for stores and products nearest to you

Until relatively recently, superfoods - in any form - have been enjoyed mainly by a small niche market of fans who stumbled across them, or had them recommended by a friend or family member. In the last few years, more supermarkets have begun putting their toe in the water by offering a small line of dried superfood products, which often seem to be located in an obscure corner of the supermarket.

Slowly but surely, superfoods are entering the mainstream consciousness; most people have heard the word 'superfoods' on television, or mentioned somewhere, but they haven't tried them and are probably still sceptical. Even if they *are* contemplating trying superfoods, they may not know where to start.

Supermarkets that *do* carry a selection of dried superfoods, may not carry every single one of the ones that we use in our recipes, and you'll probably need to ask an assistant where they are.

Most of the products we use should be available in your local Health Food or Organic Store. Stocking of certain ones may differ according to local regional differences and tastes. We recommend, using your phonebook to ring around and check first, before you trudge around town. Most health food businesses have a website, and checking this out first will save you time and shoe leather.

Donna sells her own personally blended superfood products 'exclusively online' to New Zealand and Australian customers, and there are probably similar online superfood stores in your country or region. Google is your friend; just try typing in the name of the product you're looking for and your location and hopefully you'll find what you're looking for nearby.

Since Donna's business is solely based down-under, the high cost of shipping generally makes it impractical and prohibitive to offer her products further afield than New Zealand and Australia.

If you live in the US, we recommend ordering via Amazon.com, if you don't have a preferred local supplier. Amazon makes it very easy. If you are based in the USA, it makes sense because ALL of the products we use are available on Amazon. You can order from the comfort of your own home, and their shipping costs are very reasonable within the US.

To help you choose from Amazon's huge range, Donna has selected a comparable matching superfood product on Amazon that she believes to be highest quality equivalent to her own range*. (See pg. 62 – 'Superfoods Descriptions + Info')

* NOTE: Because we don't *control* these products, we can't guarantee
  that all the Amazon links will continue to remain valid in the future.

If you don't want to shop online and you don't find a good local supplier on your first try, it may be a matter of persevering until you come across one you like.

We hope this advice helps you find a reliable source of superfoods locally. If not, reach out to us on Facebook and we'll try to help.

* * *

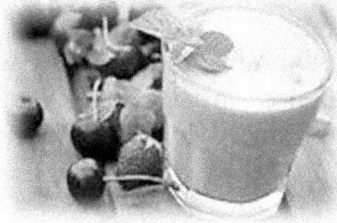

"Berries are rich in vitamin C, as well as vitamins A, B1, B2, B3 and E and also calcium, magnesium, zinc and copper."

-Donna.

Conclusion

Try our 'Chocolate Pudding' Challenge ...

If you haven't tried superfoods yet I'm sure you're asking yourself, 'Will superfoods *really* help me be healthier and feel better?'

It's a good question. So, what's our answer?

It's tempting just to say, YES, because they worked for me! But, for a more 'nutrient-dense' answer, let's look a little deeper at the quality of the food produced by our 'modern' food production methods.

Let's consider the vital relationship between our modern diet and our health. The steady and observable decline in health and rise of chronic conditions such as allergies, asthma, and skin conditions in western countries over the last 60-100 years is generally agreed by scientists and medical experts to be in large part attributable to changes in our diet.

What about other factors, like exercise?

The other biggest factor in this decline is undoubtedly the increasing trend of employment moving from outdoor, physical work to more sedentary occupations.

This takes us away from the best natural source of vitamin D (the sun) and regular exposure to rare, but necessary, elements such as selenium (from soil). This trend weakens our muscles (including the heart) and also weakens our immune system (from lack of exposure to bacterial challenges). It also slows our metabolism, decreasing its efficiency to burn fats and other harmful elements in our food that would have, under our previously vigorous outdoor lifestyle, been burned up, utilised, or expelled by our bodies.

Can it all be attributed to our modern lifestyle?

The factors we touched on in the previous paragraph, combined with the fact that our lungs (with subsequent flow-on to our blood streams) are now more likely to be sucking in stale, unhealthy air (often) full of mould spores and germs into our bodies - rather than fresh air on a regular basis, show that our modern lifestyle is far less healthy than that of our grandparents or great-grandparents.

They probably worked outside and ate a lot of fresh, uncontaminated produce that they grew themselves, or at least had easy access to, in a way that most modern city-dwellers do not. What most modern city-dwellers *do* have easy access to, are lots of highly processed, packaged, nutrient-poor foods; full of added sugars, salts and fats; coloured and chemically enhanced to 'look' fresh. Yum, yum.

Ironically, advancements in medicine are keeping increasingly unhealthy, chronically sick people alive longer, to enjoy a poorer quality of life. That's our very broad overview of the modern diet and lifestyle in most 'western' countries; it seems to us to be becoming the reality for more and more people every day.

Thanks to the Internet, a growing awareness of these issues is spreading around the world and is leading to the strong realisation that we need to change our unhealthy eating lifestyles. We believe the rapid growth of the superfood community worldwide is also evidence of that. Unfortunately, *cost* shuts many out from healthier food and nutrition alternatives, including superfoods.

We've noticed the use of 'hype' in the marketing of certain 'trendy' superfoods...

Sadly, there are always some greedy or unscrupulous (or maybe even a few genuine, but ignorant) marketers who are willing to make extravagant claims around a particular 'currently trendy' superfood, in order to exploit the gullible, the vulnerable, and sometimes desperate people hoping for some miraculous cure for a serious health condition.

While superfoods can be helpful to many health conditions and will support the body in its fight to repair and heal itself, they're best used long-term as part of a healthy lifestyle and balanced diet, for general health. They are unlikely to produce a miraculous effect on someone in the last stages of a major or life-threatening illness. Please consult your licensed medical practitioner for advice if you, or a loved one, are thinking of incorporating superfoods as part of a treatment program for any such condition.

However, for most people, there are many compelling reasons to consider adding superfoods to your diet. While sceptics remain, it is hard to deny the increasing wealth of anecdotal evidence for the benefits of incorporating superfoods into one's diet.

On the simple principle of 'rubbish in, rubbish out' it logically makes sense that putting natural, raw, organic foods into our bodies will generally lead to a better functioning bodily system than consuming nutrient-poor, non-natural foods full of chemicals and additives, as well as added sugars and fats.

The superfood *trend* tells us ...

There seems to be an emerging 'awareness' among like-minded people around the world who are choosing to eat better, think better and feel better by eating healthy, nutrient-rich foods. These are the people Donna has dubbed 'superfoodies'; she coined this term to describe those who both love and are very knowledgeable about good food (foodies), but who also consider superfoods among the wisest and best ingredients to incorporate into the creation of good food.

* * *

Try our 'Chocolate Pudding' Challenge ...

Isn't the proof always *in* the pudding?

So, why not give superfoods a try?

In our experience, most people find, after adding superfoods to their regular diet (often by simply replacing breakfast with a superfood smoothie), that they feel more energetic; they start noticing improvements in, or even the total elimination of, minor health irritations; that they're losing weight, or maintaining a healthy weight; and generally feeling more sustained and balanced.

Elsewhere in this book we've included some of the testimonials and stories (See pg.66) that Donna gets regularly from people using her 'Superfoodies' products. You can find tons more completely independent testimonials if you Google, 'testimonials about superfoods' (for example), to find loads more people reporting similar superfoods experiences all around the world.

You'll find all 21 recipes in this book delicious and easy-to-make, as well as being good for you and your loved ones.

We hope you enjoy them *all* and find yourself reaping the healthy rewards of superfoods, very soon.

 - Donna & Kay.

PS. Don't forget you're not alone; there's a whole community of 'super foodies' travelling with you.

Please reach out to us via Facebook or email, if you need help making the recipes, or any other superfoods advice. We look forward to hearing about your journey.

FOLLOW Donna on Facebook :: Facebook.com/SuperFoodies

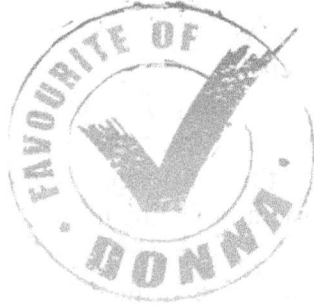

Still not sure which recipe to try first ?

We recommend you start with one of Donna's
Top 3 'Tick Start' recipes. They're the
ones with this 'tick' icon.

Find them on these pages:

1. **Strawberry Oats** → TRY ME on pg.14
2. **Berry Buckwheat Porridge** → TRY ME on pg.10
3. **Strawberry Chocolate Mousse** → TRY ME on pg.46

Why not try one tonight?

But *before* you rush off to the kitchen …

The End

Except

Donna Davidson and Kay Wood

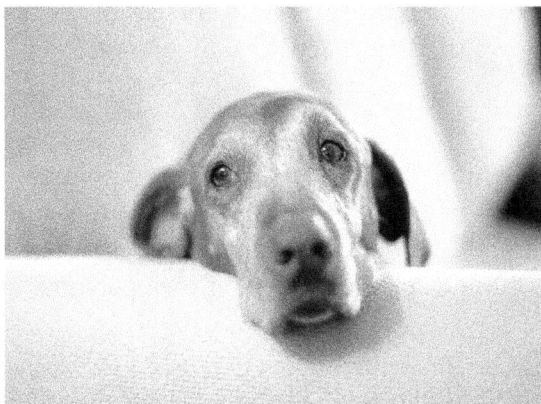

To thank *you* sincerely for buying our book!

We really appreciate it.

Would you be kind enough to help us
make our next book *even* better ?

Please take a few minutes to give us
your honest REVIEW on Amazon.com

Thanks so much!

Donna & Kay

Recipe Diary

IT'S OK TO PLAY WITH YOUR FOOD!

Have superfood fun being 'experimental'...

Why this Recipe Diary?

Donna's recipes are designed around a base of 'core' ingredients that she has carefully balanced to deliver *nutritional punch* and flavour.

They are intentionally built from a combination of 'dried superfoods' and healthy fresh ingredients that allow you to experiment around these core ingredients, to create your own variations, adapting each recipe to your own personal tastes.

* Note: Smoothie recipes particularly lend themselves to adaption because of the frequency of using them (daily). Finding alternatives for certain ingredients also helps when you encounter seasonal un-availability of fresh ingredients.

One day, Donna intends to release a book which specifically isolates the (absolutely essential) *core* ingredients in her recipes and highlighting which *optional* ingredients may be exchanged with others; without losing any of the targeted benefits and nutritional value.

But until that book comes out, why not conduct your own experiments to see what variations on Donna's recipes will work for you? Obviously, not *every* ingredient change will work, so you may have a misfire or two, but that's all part of the fun!

Donna does a lot of *experimenting* herself, and brings a lot of existing knowledge and years of experience to guide her, but balancing nutritional content with appropriate flavour combinations can be tricky sometimes. That's why 'tried and true' combinations are great starting points. Sometimes you may have to compromise on one thing in order to retain another. Some great flavour combinations are not necessarily as healthy or beneficial as others that may be less agreeable to the taste buds. The ideal result, of course, is to achieve the perfect balance of both.

Since Donna has done most of the work with these recipes, she recommends that you try your own experiments to find out if your own personal favourite will work - once you've given the originals a fair go, of course!

The best way to do this would be to change out only *one* of the fresh ingredients each time you make the recipe, and see what you think. Is it good? Does it taste terrible? Does it work with the other ingredients? Once you think you're on the right track, you could try adding one or two more new flavours with additional fresh ingredients. Don't forget to try some nuts or seeds, too.

Donna recommends you don't go 'overboard' with adding 'too many' new ingredients, because your body can only absorb so many good things in one go. You may be just wasting your money, time - and ingredients. That's why it's best to start with one change, then proceed up to two or three in total. If your experiments work, that will give you sufficient new options, without going crazy!

There will also be plenty of times when adaption, or experimentation, is absolutely necessary!

Sometimes this will be forced upon you by seasonal un-availability of fresh fruit and vegetables, or by the fact you simply forgot to replenish your pantry! It happens to the best of us. You've been busy rushing around all week and finally that birthday party or gathering of family or friends is suddenly upon you. You planned to delight everybody with your amazingly healthy chocolate treats, but when you rush to the pantry… shock, horror!… some key ingredient of a recipe is missing! Maybe more than one. You've got literally, 'no time' to replenish them, so you're forced to adapt and try to find something new to replace what is missing.

That's a great reason, for trying a few 'experiments', with ingredient variations, long *before* you find yourself in that dire situation.

It's not such a daunting prospect if you already *know* that certain flavour combinations are successful, and you already understand how to 'balance' different flavour 'profiles' against each other. 'Tried and true' is only that way because, back down the track, someone tried experimenting until they got it right! You don't want find yourself experimenting on your guests, and hoping it's not a disaster!

So, after you've given the existing recipes a good and thorough try-out (which should keep you busy for a while), use these workbook pages to keep track of your 'experiments'. Record the details here.

Don't just rely on your memory ...

Especially in those moments of panic, when you need to quickly throw something together at short notice. It's much better to come back to your notes, in your very own handwriting, in this section of the book, and *confirm* what your memory is telling you.

So, now you see how it works, when you are ready, here is ...

A good place to Start

How to use this Diary:

These steps are suggestions only. If you prefer your own way, that's ok.

1. Enjoy - experimenting with Donna's Recipes.

2. Record - your results in this Diary.

3. Change-out - <u>one</u> recipe ingredient at a time.

   (Fresh ingredients are easiest.)

4. Decide - if you like the change. If you do, you can

   either stop ... or continue.

5. Change / or Add - up to 2 more ingredients.

6. Record - your changes, and your thoughts on the

   results in the 'Notes' section.

7. Rate - your experiment out of 7. Also circle either:

   Yes – No – Maybe

Happy experimenting! Have *lots* of fun.

Experiment #1

Recipe Notes:

Don't rely on your memory! Fill in *all* the details here and you'll always know exactly what you did - and if it worked or not.

Date: ....

Recipe Name: ....…....….

Change #1: _____

Change #2: _____

Change #3: _____

*My Results: _____

_____

_____

_____

Rate the Result: [Circle the number you believe to be the fairest.]

1   2   3   4   5   6   7

* <u>Don't</u> forget to record what you learn about different flavour combos. Could the new flavour work in a different recipe, or combination? Could it work with the addition of a balancing flavour/or flavours? If any other *inspired* ideas occur as you go, note them down for future experiments.

Circle one: YES!   NO!   MAYBE?

Experiment #2

Recipe Notes:

Don't rely on your memory! Fill in *all* the details here and you'll always know exactly what you did - and if it worked or not.

Date: ....

Recipe Name: ....……........

Change #1:

Change #2:

Change #3:

*My Results:

Rate the Result: [Circle the number you believe to be the fairest.]

1   2   3   4   5   6   7

* Don't forget to record what you learn about different flavour combos. Could the new flavour work in a different recipe, or combination? Could it work with the addition of a balancing flavour/or flavours? If any other *inspired* ideas occur as you go, note them down for future experiments.

Circle one: YES!   NO!   MAYBE?

Experiment #3

Recipe Notes:

Don't rely on your memory! Fill in *all* the details here and you'll always know exactly what you did - and if it worked or not.

Date: ....

Recipe Name: ....

Change #1: ....

Change #2: ....

Change #3: ....

*My Results: ....

....

....

....

Rate the Result: [Circle the number you believe to be the fairest.]

1   2   3   4   5   6   7

* Don't forget to record what you learn about different flavour combos. Could the new flavour work in a different recipe, or combination? Could it work with the addition of a balancing flavour/or flavours? If any other *inspired* ideas occur as you go, note them down for future experiments.

Circle one: YES!   NO!   MAYBE?

Experiment #4

Recipe Notes:

Don't rely on your memory! Fill in *all* the details here and you'll always know exactly what you did - and if it worked or not.

Date: ....

Recipe Name: ....…..……

Change #1:

Change #2:

Change #3:

*My Results:

Rate the Result: [Circle the number you believe to be the fairest.]

1   2   3   4   5   6   7

* <u>Don't</u> forget to record what you learn about different flavour combos. Could the new flavour work in a different recipe, or combination? Could it work with the addition of a balancing flavour/or flavours? If any other *inspired* ideas occur as you go, note them down for future experiments.

Circle one: YES!   NO!   MAYBE?

Experiment #5

Recipe Notes:

Don't rely on your memory! Fill in *all* the details here and you'll always know exactly what you did - and if it worked or not.

Date: ....

Recipe Name: ....……......

Change #1: _____

Change #2: _____

Change #3: _____

*My Results: _____

_____

_____

_____

Rate the Result: [Circle the number you believe to be the fairest.]

1   2   3   4   5   6   7

* <u>Don't</u> forget to record what you learn about different flavour combos. Could the new flavour work in a different recipe, or combination? Could it work with the addition of a balancing flavour/or flavours? If any other *inspired* ideas occur as you go, note them down for future experiments.

Circle one: YES!   NO!   MAYBE?

Experiment #6

Recipe Notes:

Don't rely on your memory! Fill in *all* the details here and you'll always know exactly what you did - and if it worked or not.

Date: ....

Recipe Name: ....…......

Change #1: _____

Change #2: _____

Change #3: _____

*My Results: _____

_____

_____

_____

Rate the Result: [Circle the number you believe to be the fairest.]

1   2   3   4   5   6   7

* Don't forget to record what you learn about different flavour combos. Could the new flavour work in a different recipe, or combination? Could it work with the addition of a balancing flavour/or flavours? If any other *inspired* ideas occur as you go, note them down for future experiments.

Circle one: YES!   NO!   MAYBE?

Experiment #7

Recipe Notes:

Don't rely on your memory! Fill in *all* the details here and you'll always know exactly what you did - and if it worked or not.

Date: ....

Recipe Name: ....…........

Change #1: _____

Change #2: _____

Change #3: _____

*My Results: _____

_____

_____

_____

Rate the Result: [Circle the number you believe to be the fairest.]

1   2   3   4   5   6   7

* <u>Don't</u> forget to record what you learn about different flavour combos. Could the new flavour work in a different recipe, or combination? Could it work with the addition of a balancing flavour/or flavours? If any other *inspired* ideas occur as you go, note them down for future experiments.

Circle one: YES!   NO!   MAYBE?

Experiment #8

Recipe Notes:

Don't rely on your memory! Fill in *all* the details here and you'll always know exactly what you did - and if it worked or not.

Date: ....

Recipe Name: ....……........

Change #1:

Change #2:

Change #3:

*My Results:

Rate the Result: [Circle the number you believe to be the fairest.]

1   2   3   4   5   6   7

* <u>Don't</u> forget to record what you learn about different flavour combos. Could the new flavour work in a different recipe, or combination? Could it work with the addition of a balancing flavour/or flavours? If any other *inspired* ideas occur as you go, note them down for future experiments.

Circle one: YES!   NO!   MAYBE?

Experiment #9

Recipe Notes:

Don't rely on your memory! Fill in *all* the details here and you'll always know exactly what you did - and if it worked or not.

Date: ....

Recipe Name: ....

Change #1: _____

Change #2: _____

Change #3: _____

*My Results: _____

_____

_____

_____

Rate the Result: [Circle the number you believe to be the fairest.]

1   2   3   4   5   6   7

* <u>Don't</u> forget to record what you learn about different flavour combos. Could the new flavour work in a different recipe, or combination? Could it work with the addition of a balancing flavour/or flavours? If any other *inspired* ideas occur as you go, note them down for future experiments.

Circle one: YES!   NO!   MAYBE?

Experiment #10

Recipe Notes:

Don't rely on your memory! Fill in *all* the details here and you'll always know exactly what you did - and if it worked or not.

Date: ....

Recipe Name: ....

Change #1:

Change #2:

Change #3:

*My Results:

Rate the Result: [Circle the number you believe to be the fairest.]

1   2   3   4   5   6   7

* <u>Don't</u> forget to record what you learn about different flavour combos. Could the new flavour work in a different recipe, or combination? Could it work with the addition of a balancing flavour/or flavours? If any other *inspired* ideas occur as you go, note them down for future experiments.

Circle one: YES!   NO!   MAYBE?

Experiment #11

Recipe Notes:

Don't rely on your memory! Fill in *all* the details here and you'll always know exactly what you did - and if it worked or not.

Date: ....

Recipe Name: ....……

Change #1: ....

Change #2: ....

Change #3: ....

*My Results: ....

....

....

....

Rate the Result: [Circle the number you believe to be the fairest.]

1   2   3   4   5   6   7

* <u>Don't</u> forget to record what you learn about different flavour combos. Could the new flavour work in a different recipe, or combination? Could it work with the addition of a balancing flavour/or flavours? If any other *inspired* ideas occur as you go, note them down for future experiments.

Circle one: YES!   NO!   MAYBE?

Experiment #12

Recipe Notes:

Don't rely on your memory! Fill in *all* the details here and you'll always know exactly what you did - and if it worked or not.

Date: ....

Recipe Name: ....

Change #1:

Change #2:

Change #3:

*My Results:

Rate the Result: [Circle the number you believe to be the fairest.]

1   2   3   4   5   6   7

* Don't forget to record what you learn about different flavour combos. Could the new flavour work in a different recipe, or combination? Could it work with the addition of a balancing flavour/or flavours? If any other *inspired* ideas occur as you go, note them down for future experiments.

Circle one: YES!   NO!   MAYBE?

Experiment #13

Recipe Notes:

Don't rely on your memory! Fill in *all* the details here and you'll always know exactly what you did - and if it worked or not.

Date: ....

Recipe Name: ....…......

Change #1: ....

Change #2: ....

Change #3: ....

*My Results: ....

....

....

....

Rate the Result: [Circle the number you believe to be the fairest.]

1   2   3   4   5   6   7

* <u>Don't</u> forget to record what you learn about different flavour combos. Could the new flavour work in a different recipe, or combination? Could it work with the addition of a balancing flavour/or flavours? If any other *inspired* ideas occur as you go, note them down for future experiments.

Circle one: YES!   NO!   MAYBE?

Experiment #14

Recipe Notes:

Don't rely on your memory! Fill in *all* the details here and you'll always know exactly what you did - and if it worked or not.

Date: ....

Recipe Name: ....…..……

Change #1: ....

Change #2: ....

Change #3: ....

*My Results: ....

....

....

....

Rate the Result: [Circle the number you believe to be the fairest.]

1   2   3   4   5   6   7

* <u>Don't</u> forget to record what you learn about different flavour combos. Could the new flavour work in a different recipe, or combination? Could it work with the addition of a balancing flavour/or flavours? If any other *inspired* ideas occur as you go, note them down for future experiments.

Circle one: YES!   NO!   MAYBE?

Experiment #15

Recipe Notes:

Don't rely on your memory! Fill in *all* the details here and you'll always know exactly what you did - and if it worked or not.

Date: ....

Recipe Name: ....…..……

Change #1:

Change #2:

Change #3:

*My Results:

Rate the Result: [Circle the number you believe to be the fairest.]

1   2   3   4   5   6   7

* Don't forget to record what you learn about different flavour combos. Could the new flavour work in a different recipe, or combination? Could it work with the addition of a balancing flavour/or flavours? If any other *inspired* ideas occur as you go, note them down for future experiments.

Circle one: YES!   NO!   MAYBE?

Experiment #16

Recipe Notes:

Don't rely on your memory! Fill in *all* the details here and you'll always know exactly what you did - and if it worked or not.

Date: ....

Recipe Name: ....……......

Change #1:

Change #2:

Change #3:

*My Results:

Rate the Result: [Circle the number you believe to be the fairest.]

1   2   3   4   5   6   7

* <u>Don't</u> forget to record what you learn about different flavour combos. Could the new flavour work in a different recipe, or combination? Could it work with the addition of a balancing flavour/or flavours? If any other *inspired* ideas occur as you go, note them down for future experiments.

Circle one: YES!   NO!   MAYBE?

Experiment #17

Recipe Notes:

Don't rely on your memory! Fill in *all* the details here and you'll always know exactly what you did - and if it worked or not.

Date: ....

Recipe Name: ....

Change #1:

Change #2:

Change #3:

*My Results:

Rate the Result: [Circle the number you believe to be the fairest.]

1   2   3   4   5   6   7

* <u>Don't</u> forget to record what you learn about different flavour combos. Could the new flavour work in a different recipe, or combination? Could it work with the addition of a balancing flavour/or flavours? If any other *inspired* ideas occur as you go, note them down for future experiments.

Circle one: YES!   NO!   MAYBE?

Experiment #18

Recipe Notes:

Don't rely on your memory! Fill in *all* the details here and you'll always know exactly what you did - and if it worked or not.

Date: ....

Recipe Name: ....

Change #1:

Change #2:

Change #3:

*My Results:

Rate the Result: [Circle the number you believe to be the fairest.]

1   2   3   4   5   6   7

* Don't forget to record what you learn about different flavour combos. Could the new flavour work in a different recipe, or combination? Could it work with the addition of a balancing flavour/or flavours? If any other *inspired* ideas occur as you go, note them down for future experiments.

Circle one: YES!   NO!   MAYBE?

Experiment #19

Recipe Notes:

Don't rely on your memory! Fill in *all* the details here and you'll always know exactly what you did - and if it worked or not.

Date: ....

Recipe Name: ....

Change #1:

Change #2:

Change #3:

*My Results:

Rate the Result: [Circle the number you believe to be the fairest.]

1   2   3   4   5   6   7

* <u>Don't</u> forget to record what you learn about different flavour combos. Could the new flavour work in a different recipe, or combination? Could it work with the addition of a balancing flavour/or flavours? If any other *inspired* ideas occur as you go, note them down for future experiments.

Circle one: YES!   NO!   MAYBE?

Experiment #20

Recipe Notes:

Don't rely on your memory! Fill in *all* the details here and you'll always know exactly what you did - and if it worked or not.

Date: ....

Recipe Name: ....……......

Change #1: ....

Change #2: ....

Change #3: ....

*My Results: ....

....

....

....

Rate the Result: [Circle the number you believe to be the fairest.]

1   2   3   4   5   6   7

* Don't forget to record what you learn about different flavour combos. Could the new flavour work in a different recipe, or combination? Could it work with the addition of a balancing flavour/or flavours? If any other *inspired* ideas occur as you go, note them down for future experiments.

Circle one: YES!   NO!   MAYBE?

Experiment #21

Recipe Notes:

Don't rely on your memory! Fill in *all* the details here and you'll always know exactly what you did - and if it worked or not.

Date: ....

Recipe Name: ....…..…....

Change #1:

Change #2:

Change #3:

*My Results:

Rate the Result: [Circle the number you believe to be the fairest.]

1   2   3   4   5   6   7

* <u>Don't</u> forget to record what you learn about different flavour combos. Could the new flavour work in a different recipe, or combination? Could it work with the addition of a balancing flavour/or flavours? If any other *inspired* ideas occur as you go, note them down for future experiments.

Circle one: YES!   NO!   MAYBE?

Want <u>more</u> recipe diary pages?

You could just *photocopy* the pages of this book … if you don't mind loose pages floating around - that can easily get misplaced.

But, if you'd rather enjoy the convenience of having them all neatly bound together in one book, this 105 page 'Mini Recipe Diary' maybe what you are looking for …

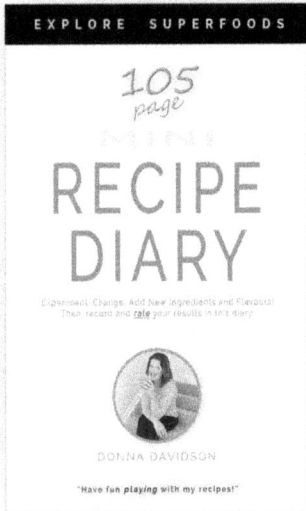

Companion Diary to Donna's Recipe Books:

'Mini Recipe Diary' – 105 pages*

Change, vary, experiment with Donna's recipes! Record and rate the results here in your very own recipe diary. You'll always know which changes you loved and which never to repeat – especially when you have guests!

ONLY US.$9 – print book
Order now from Amazon.com

* *More sizes will be available soon.*

* * *

Amazon Link: Mini Recipe Diary
www.amazon.com/dp/047337966X

WHERE TO START?

TRY ME!

Don't forget…

1. Your 3 <u>Free</u> Bonus Superfood Recipes!

Type this into your Internet browser:
superfoodies.co.nz/book3free

2. Our other books…

Book #1: 21 Best Superfood Cacao Recipes
Go here: www.amazon.com/dp/B0178USZ88

Book #2: 21 Best Superfood Smoothie Recipes
Go here: www.amazon.com/dp/B01J73OAKG

3. You can help us – with an honest <u>review</u> …

We write our books with *you* in mind. Please take 5 minutes to give us your honest REVIEW on Amazon. Tell us what you <u>like</u> about our book(s) – and where we can <u>improve</u> for you, in future editions.

Review here > www.amazon.com/dp/B01LWJLKOD

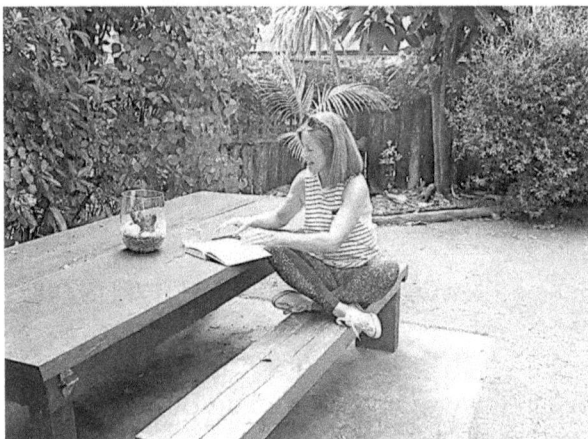

Dreaming of writing your own book?

Many people spend years wanting to write a book but never do ... Why?

How did _we_ manage it?

We found a great online writers school, called 'Self-Publishing School'. They provided coaching, training, support, and a step-by-step plan to publishing our first book in 90 days, guaranteed.

They also showed us how to format, upload, and successfully market our book. They involved us in a supportive Facebook community of fellow writers who gave immediate feedback and positive advice all along the way. We had a great experience, and our first two books made it to number #1 on Amazon, so we happily commend SPS to you.

If you believe you have a book in you, but need a little help giving birth to it, check out the Self-Publishing School at the link below:

Self-Publishing School -
http://superfoodies.co.nz/sps

PHOTO Opposite: Donna relaxing in her garden in Ohope Beach, New Zealand.

Still turning pages?

Why?

Are you expecting a big …

Surprise!

EXTRA BONUS RECIPE

* * *

Healthy Breakfast Muesli

This Maca muesli will support your thyroid and the high antioxidant content will support your general health.

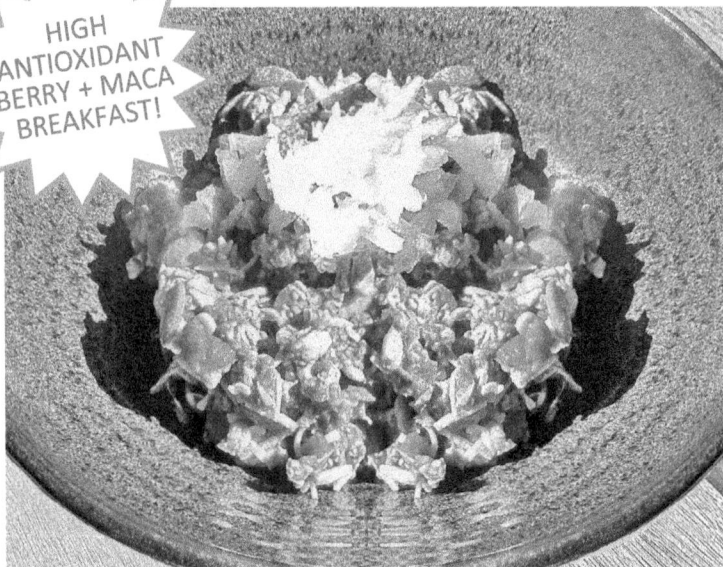

HIGH ANTIOXIDANT BERRY + MACA BREAKFAST!

Maca Bircher Muesli

Serving size: makes 2 servings
Time to make: 5 mins + soaking time

Ingredients

2 teaspoons maqui berry powder

2 teaspoons maca powder

½ cup organic rolled oats

1 teaspoon chia seeds

1 tablespoon desiccated coconut

1 tablespoon dried goji berries

1 teaspoon sunflower seeds

1 teaspoon pumpkin seeds

1 tablespoon chopped nuts - almonds / or your choice of nuts

1 tablespoon chopped dates

1 teaspoon vanilla extract

1 cup liquid - water / coconut water / or almond milk

Method

1. Place all dry ingredients in a bowl and mix well.
2. Add your liquid of choice to the vanilla extract and soak overnight or if you forget to soak overnight 1 hr can be enough.
3. To garnish when ready to eat, stir through some grated apple / pear / or whatever appeals to you.
4. Top with coconut cream or yoghurt.

* Notes:

If you like this maca recipe you can make up a large jar of the dry ingredients and store it so that you only need to place a cup of dry ingredients in a bowl then add the liquid to soak.

Maca supports healthy thyroid function.

Also play with the ingredients; you can substitute maca for lucuma, or you can use both!

Some people find maca difficult to tolerate and may experience minor stomach cramps or nausea - although this is not common. I've used a full tablespoon from the start and had no problems at all. However, everybody is different so you may want to try a little first and see if you can tolerate it well. I hope so, because I love maca and I don't want you to miss out on this great superfood.

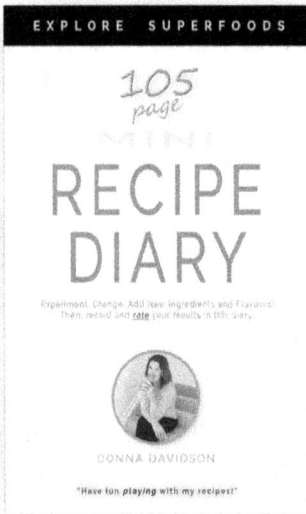

* * *

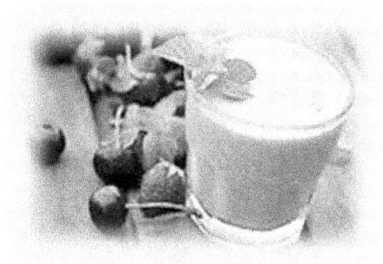

"Berries carry high levels of antioxidants that are essential to keep our cells healthy and free from life threatening diseases."

–Donna.

YOUR KIDS WILL LOVE THIS!

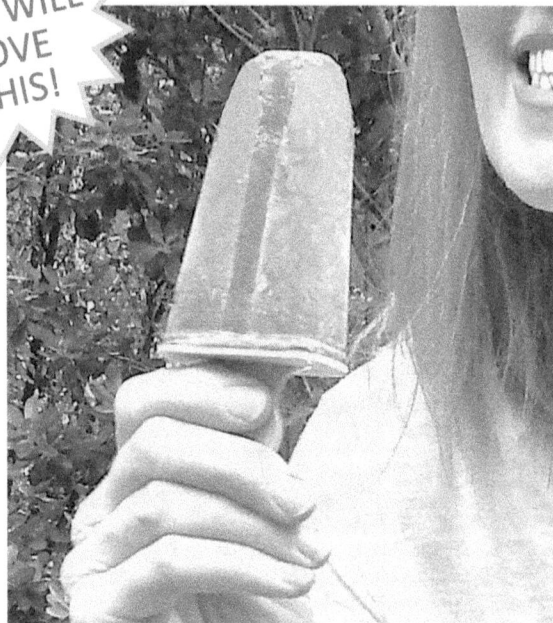

Surprise your kids this summer…

Turn my superfood smoothies into delicious, <u>healthy popsicles</u>!

Your kids will love them! They're yummy, flavour-packed 'superfood popsicles' - ideal for hot summer days.

Or *anytime* you feel like a cool treat.

They're ridiculously *easy* to make ...

Just pour your liquid smoothies into popsicle molds and 'pop' them in your freezer overnight, or until solid. Simple as 1,2,3.

1. Make your favourite smoothie.

2. Pour into a popsicle mold.

3. Place in freezer until solid.

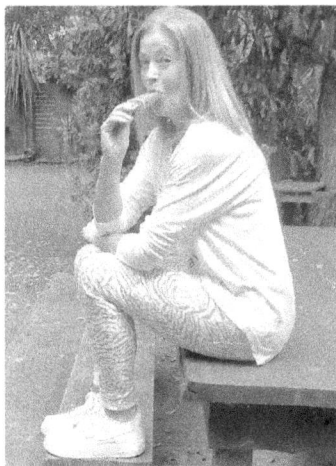

Then, treat your family and friends to the healthiest, tastiest popsicle they've probably ever eaten!

Kids love berry and fruit smoothie popsicles best - because they're flavour-packed and super delicious. And they won't even know they are healthy! These popsicles are a great way to avoid the sugary, unhealthy ice-creams and cordial-based alternatives.

Where can you find popsicle molds?

Popsicle molds are cheap – from $10 to $20 US – and can be purchased from a zillion retailers from Walmart to Kmart.

You can order them online from Amazon, too.

For example, below is just one we found on Amazon with a quick search for 'popsicle molds'.

Here's the Amazon link to the above:
www.amazon.com/gp/product/B0002IBJOG

However, once you go there you will see links to a wide array of other choices below that product. Or, just do your own search for 'popsicle molds' in Amazon's search box.

Here are just a *few* different kinds of
popsicle molds available ...

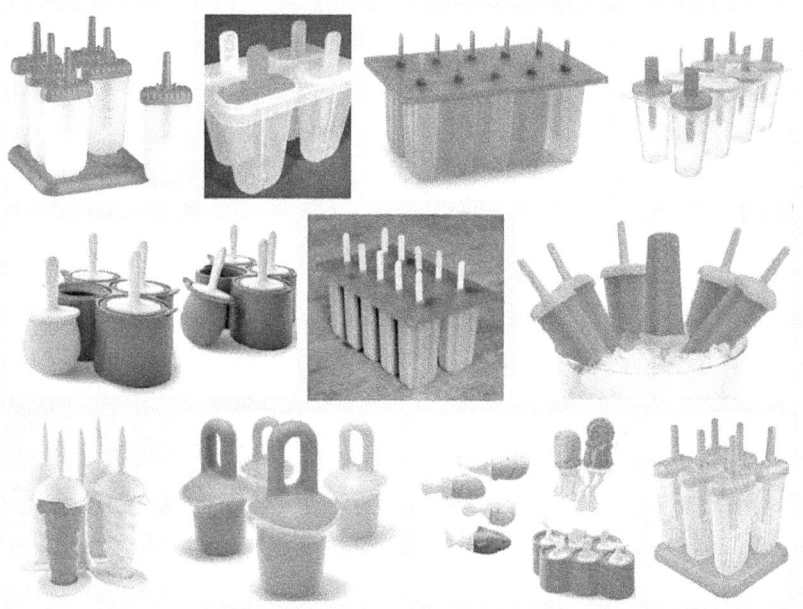

The screen-shot above shows a small selection of the different
popsicle molds on the market. These are from Amazom.com but
you can find a huge variety at other retailers, like Walmart.

Popsicle molds come in lots of colourful shapes and sizes that
your kids will love. Plus, they'll make your 'healthy
popsicles' even *more* fun to eat!

Be aware:

Some molds come with sticks attached (silicone/plastic) and
some use wooden sticks you'll need to buy more of
when the supplied ones run out.

* * *

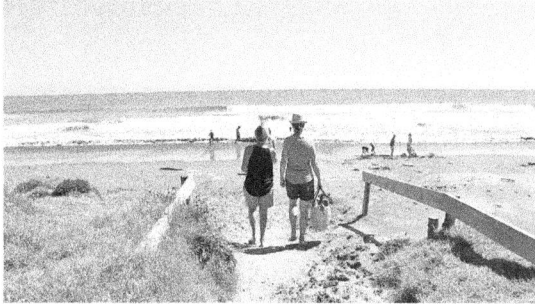

Bye, for now,

We're off to the beach.
See you in our next book.

-Donna & Kay.

End.

Books by Donna & Kay

The Discover Superfoods Series — *by* Donna Davidson and Kay Wood.

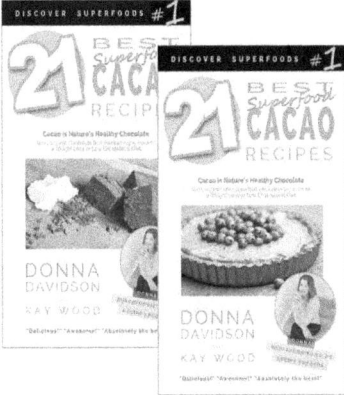

KINDLE / eBook
Discover Superfoods Book #1
21 Best Superfood Cacao Recipes
Available on Amazon.

PRINT BOOK
Discover Superfoods Book #1
21 Best Superfood Cacao Recipes
Available on Amazon.

* * * * * * * * * * * * *

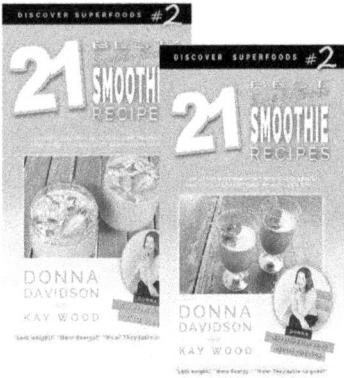

KINDLE / eBook
Discover Superfoods Book #2
21 Best Superfood Smoothie Recipes
Available on Amazon

PRINT BOOK
Discover Superfoods Book #2
21 Best Superfood Smoothie Recipes
Available on Amazon

* * * * * * * * * * * * *

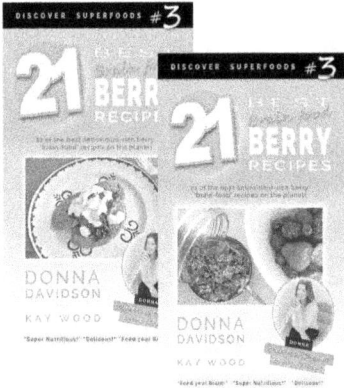

KINDLE / eBook
Discover Superfoods Book #3
21 Best Berry Brain-food Recipes
Available on Amazon

PRINT BOOK
Discover Superfoods Book #3
21 Best Berry Brain-food Recipes
Available on Amazon

135

The Secret
to better health?

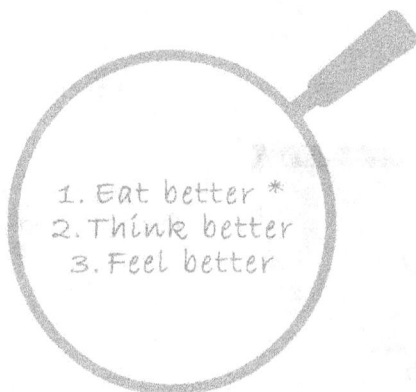

1. Eat better *
2. Think better
3. Feel better

* "Good food is better _medicine_ than medicine. If you enjoy the privilege of being able to choose
to eat better, you are among the lucky ones. Make that choice today and save
on your future medical bills, mental anguish, physical pain, and years
of living with a lower quality of life than you needed to."

- D&K.

www.ingramcontent.com/pod-product-compliance
Lightning Source LLC
Chambersburg PA
CBHW050131280326
41933CB00010B/1334